The Tibetan Yogas of Dream and Sleep

Books by Tenzin Wangyal Rinpoche

Awakening the Luminous Mind
Awakening the Sacred Body
Healing with Form, Energy, and Light
Spontaneous Creativity: Meditations for Manifesting Your Positive Qualities
Tibetan Sound Healing
The True Source of Healing: How the Ancient Tibetan Practice of Soul Retrieval Can Transform and Enrich Your Life
Unbounded Wholeness: Dzogchen, Bon and, the Logic of the Nonconceptual (with Anne Carolyn Klein)
Wonders of the Natural Mind

The Tibetan Yogas of Dream and Sleep

Practices for Awakening

Revised Edition

TENZIN WANGYAL RINPOCHE

Edited by Mark Dahlby
Foreword by the Dalai Lama

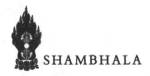 SHAMBHALA

Shambhala Publications, Inc.
2129 13th Street
Boulder, Colorado 80302
www.shambhala.com

Cover photo: StockByM/iStock
Cover design: Daniel Urban-Brown

9 8 7 6 5 4 3 2 1

Second Edition
Printed in the United States of America

Shambhala Publications makes every effort to print on
acid-free, recycled paper.

Shambhala Publications is distributed worldwide by
Penguin Random House, Inc., and its subsidiaries.

LIBRARY OF CONGRESS CATALOGING-IN-PUBLICATION DATA
Names: Wangyal, Tenzin, author. | Dahlby, Mark, editor.
Title: The Tibetan yogas of dream and sleep: practices for awakening /
Tenzin Wangyal Rinpoche; edited by Mark Dahlby.
Description: Boulder, Colorado: Shambhala, [2022] |
Includes bibliographical references.
Identifiers: LCCN 2021042554 | ISBN 9781611809510 (trade paperback)
Subjects: LCSH: Yoga—Bon. | Dreams—Religious aspects—
Bon (Tibetan religion) | Sleep—Religious aspects—Bon (Tibetan religion)
Classification: LCC BQ7982.2 .W36 2022 | DDC 299.5/4—dc23
LCrecord available at https://lccn.loc.gov/2021042554

This book is dedicated to Namkhai Norbu Rinpoche, who was a great inspiration in my life, both in how I teach others and in my own practice.

Contents

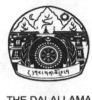

THE DALAI LAMA

Tenzin Wangyal, a geshe of Yungdrung Bön, has written a book called *The Tibetan Yogas of Dream and Sleep*. I rejoice that it has been translated into many languages, introducing the topic to many countries, primarily in the West. Because Tibetan Dharma is taking on new forms in various Western countries, it is most important in those countries to focus on the proper custom of uniting study and practice in order to establish excellent opportunities for teaching and learning the Dharma. Therefore, there is a special need for general presentations of the ground, path, and fruition, as well as the view, meditation, and action that appear in Bön's own texts. I make the aspiration that, from this point forward, this composition that points out the practices of dream and sleep will serve as a support for Bön teachings and that vast waves of benefit will arise for many people.

February 9, 2022

Editor's Preface
to the Second Edition

In 2020, early in the COVID-19 pandemic, Nikko Odiseos of Shambhala Publications sent an email to Tenzin Wangyal Rinpoche suggesting a second edition of *The Tibetan Yogas of Dream and Sleep*, perhaps with some new material or a new chapter. It grew into something more during the rewrite.

The first edition grew from oral teaching Rinpoche gave in California and New Mexico and was written over several years, starting in the midnineties. It was published by Snow Lion in 1998 and has been translated into twenty-five languages and more have been requested.

The second edition incorporates teachings given through online retreats to participants in several countries during the pandemic, in 2020 and 2021.

Tenzin Wangyal Rinpoche began teaching in the West in 1988. Since, he has taught thousands of students, both in person in many countries and, increasingly, online to reach students in different parts of the world, in different time zones, and speaking different languages. The essence of Rinpoche's teaching is Dzogchen; that has not changed. But over time, in response to his students' questions, he has adjusted how he articulates the teachings to make them clearer and more accessible. That change has been integrated into this edition. Changes from the first edition are noted if they alter the steps of a practice or need explanation. Other than correcting punctuation and word usage, no changes were made to the sleep yoga section.

The first use of most Tibetan and Sanskrit words are italicized, indicating they will be found in the improved glossary at the end of the book.

M.D.

Preface to the First Edition

A well-known saying in Tibetan states, "One should explain the lineage and history to cut doubt about the authenticity of the teaching and the transmission." Therefore, I begin this book with a short story of my life.

I was born not long after my parents fled the Chinese oppression in Tibet. Conditions were difficult, and my parents placed me in a Christian boarding school, where they hoped I would be cared for. My father was a Buddhist lama, my mother a practitioner of Bön. Sometime after, my father died. Eventually my mother remarried a man who was a Bön lama. Both he and my mother wanted me to live within my culture, so when I was ten years old, I was taken to the main Bön monastery in Dolanji, India, and ordained as a monk.

After living in the monastery for some time, I was recognized by Lopon (Head Teacher) Sangye Tenzin Rinpoche as the reincarnation of Khyungtul Rinpoche, a famous scholar, teacher, author, and meditation master. He was well known as a master astrologer. In western Tibet and northern India, he was famous as a tamer of wild spirits and was widely sought after as a healer with magical abilities. One of his sponsors was a local king of Himachal in northern India. The king and his wife, unable to bear children, asked Khyungtul Rinpoche to heal them, which he did. The son they bore and raised, Virbhadra Singh, became the 4th Chief Minister of Himachal Pradesh.

When I was thirteen, my kind root master, Lopon Sangye Tenzin, a man of great knowledge and realization, prepared to teach one of the most important and esoteric teachings in the Bön religion: the Great Perfection (Dzogchen) lineage of the Oral Transmission of Zhang Zhung (Zhang zhung nyan gyud). Even though I was still young, my stepfather visited Lopon Rinpoche and asked that I be admitted to the teachings, which would take place every day for three years. Lopon kindly agreed but asked that I, along with the other prospective students, bring him a dream from the night before the teachings were to begin so that he might determine our readiness.

Some of the students remembered no dream, which was considered a sign of obstacles. Lopon had them begin purification practices and delayed the beginning of the teaching until each student had a dream. Dreams of other students were taken as indications that they needed to do particular practices to ready themselves for the teachings—for example, doing practices that strengthened their connections to the Bön guardians.

I dreamt about a bus circumambulating my teacher's house, although there is actually no road there. In the dream, the bus conductor was my friend, and I stood beside him, handing out tickets to each person boarding the bus. The tickets were pieces of paper with the Tibetan syllable *A* written on them. That was in the second or third year of my education at Dolanji. At the time I didn't know *A* was a symbol of major significance in Dzogchen teachings.

My teacher never said anything about the dream, which was his way. He made little comment about what was good, but I was happy as long as I was allowed to go to the teachings.

It is common, in Tibetan spiritual traditions, for the dreams of students to be used by the teacher to determine if it is appropriate for a student to receive a particular teaching. Though it would be some time before I began to study and practice dream yoga, this incident was the beginning of my interest in dreams. It strongly impressed on me how greatly dream is valued in Tibetan culture and in the Bön religion, and how information from the unconscious is often of greater value than information the conscious mind can provide.

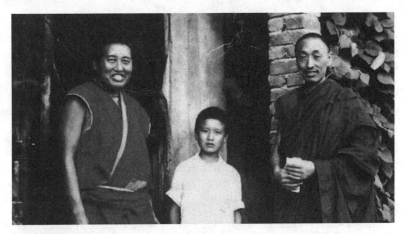

Tenzin Wangyal Rinpoche, ten years old, with H.E. Yongdzin Lopon Tenzin Namdak Rinpoche and H.H. Lungtok Tenpai Nyima, the 33rd abbot of Menri Monastery

After the three-year teaching, which included numerous meditation retreats with my fellow practitioners, as well as many retreats that I did alone, I entered the monastic Dialectic School. The program of study normally takes nine to thirteen years to complete and covers the traditional training. We were taught the common academic subjects, such as grammar, Sanskrit, poetry, astrology, and art, and we also learned the uncommon subjects: epistemology, cosmology, sutra, tantra, and Dzogchen. During monastic training, I was exposed to a number of teachings on dreams and given the transmissions needed to study and practice them. The most important teachings were based on the texts of the Zhang Zhung Nyan Gyud, the *Mother Tantra*, and Shardza Rinpoche.

I did well in the training and, when I was nineteen, was asked to begin teaching others. Around the same time, I wrote and published a summary of the biography of Lord Shenrab Miwoche, the founder of the Bön religion. Later I became the president of the Dialectic School and for four years was very involved in shaping and developing the school. In 1986, I received the *geshe* degree, the highest degree awarded in Tibetan monastic education.

In 1989, at the invitation of Namkhai Norbu Rinpoche's Dzogchen Community in Italy, I traveled to the West. I had no plans to teach but was asked to do so by members of the community. One day, I was passing out small pieces of paper to be used in a meditation on concentration. Each piece of paper had the Tibetan syllable *A* written on it. Right then the dream from fifteen years before, in which I passed out the same paper to people getting on the bus, came back to me. It was as if it hit me on the head.

I remained in the West and in 1991 was awarded a Rockefeller Fellowship to do research at Rice University. In 1993, I published my first book in the West, *The Wonders of the Natural Mind*, in which I tried to present the Great Perfection (Dzogchen) teachings in a clear and simple way. In 1994 I was given a grant from the National Endowment for the Humanities to pursue research on the logical and philosophical aspects of the Bön tradition in collaboration with Professor Anne Klein, the chair of Religious Studies at Rice University.

So my scholarly side has continued to manifest, but practice is always more important, and during all this time I have been interested in dreams and dream practice. My interest is not only theoretical. I have trusted the wisdom of my dreams, influenced from an early age by the dream experiences of my teachers and my mother and by the use of dreams in the Bön tradition, and I have been practicing dream yoga intensively during the last ten years. Every night when I get into bed, I feel freedom. The busyness of the day is over. Some nights the practice is successful, and some nights it is not. That is to be expected until the practice is very advanced. Nevertheless, I go to sleep nearly every night with the intention to accomplish dream practice. It is from my own experience with the practice, as well as from the three texts noted earlier, that the teachings in this book come.

Dream yoga is a primary support in my own practice, and this has been true for many, many masters and yogis of Tibet. For example, I have always been impressed by the life of Shardza Rinpoche, a great Tibetan master who, when he died in 1934, attained the body of light (*jalus*), a sign of full realization. During his life he had many accomplished students, wrote many important texts, and worked for the benefit of the country in which he lived. It's difficult to imagine how he could have been so productive in his external life, fulfilling the many responsibilities and long projects he undertook for the benefit of others, and still have been able to accomplish such attainment through spiritual practice. He could do this because he was not a writer for part of the day, a teacher for another part, and a practitioner for the few hours that were left. All of his life was practice, whether he was sitting in meditation, writing, teaching, or sleeping. He writes that dream practice was of central importance in his spiritual journey and integral to his attainment. This can also be true for us.

Tenzin Wangyal Rinpoche

Acknowledgments

I want to thank the people who have been instrumental in bringing this book to publication the first time. First of all, and most important, Mark Dahlby, my student and close friend, with whom I greatly enjoyed working. We spent many hours discussing different issues in cafés around Berkeley. Without him, this book would not have been possible.

Also, Steven D. Goodman, a colleague and friend, improved the manuscript through numerous good suggestions; Sue Ellis Dyer and Chris Baker made editing suggestions on an early version of the book; Sue Davis and Laura Shekerjian helped by reading a later version of the text and offering feedback; and Christine Cox of Snow Lion Publications brought her great skill as an experienced editor to the text and made it a much better book.

The photographs of the meditation and dream yoga positions in the first edition were taken by Antonio Riestra and modeled by Luz Vergara. Illustrations of the chakras were created by Monica R. Ortega. I also want to thank all those I have not named but who helped in many different ways.

For the second edition, I thank Mark Dahlby, who was again the editor. Thanks to Laura Shekerjian, who read through the manuscript and offered helpful suggestions. To Kurt Keutzer, for correcting the transliterations in the glossary and improving and clarifying entries. To Shambhala Publications, particularly Nikko Odiseos for suggesting the new edition, Tucker Foley for managing the project, and Karen Steib for improving nearly every page when she copyedited the manuscript.

The Tibetan Yogas of Dream and Sleep

Introduction

We spend a third of our life sleeping. No matter what we do, however virtuous or nonvirtuous our activities, whether we are murderers or saints, monks or libertines, every day ends the same. We shut our eyes and dissolve into darkness. We do so fearlessly, even as everything we know as "me" disappears. After a brief period, images arise, and our sense of self arises with them. We exist again in the apparently limitless world of dream. Every night we participate in these most profound mysteries, moving from one dimension of experience to another, losing our sense of self and finding it again, yet we take it all for granted. We wake in the morning and continue "real" life, but in a sense, we are still asleep and dreaming. The teachings tell us that we can continue in this deluded, dreamy state day and night, or we can wake up.

When we engage in sleep and dream yogas, we become part of a long lineage. Men and women have, for many centuries, undertaken these same practices, confronted the same doubts and obstacles that we do, and received the same benefits that we can. Many high lamas and accomplished yogis have made sleep and dream yogas primary practices and through them attained realization. Reflecting on this history and remembering the people who dedicated their lives to the teachings—our spiritual ancestors who through these teachings pass to us the fruits of their practice—will generate faith in and gratitude for the tradition.

Some Tibetan masters might find it strange that I teach these practices to Westerners who have not completed certain preliminary practices. The teachings were traditionally maintained as secret teachings, both as a sign of respect and as a protection against dilution through the misunderstanding of unprepared practitioners. They were never taught publicly or given lightly, but were reserved for individuals prepared to receive them.

The practices are no less efficacious and valuable than they ever were, but conditions in the world have changed, so I am trying something different. I hope that by teaching what is effective, openly and simply, the tradition will be better preserved, and more people will be able to benefit from it. But it is important to respect the teachings, both to protect them and to further our own practice. Please try to receive the direct transmission of these teachings from an authentic teacher. It is good to read about these yogas but better to receive the oral transmission, which creates a stronger connection with the lineage. Also, it is easy to encounter obstacles on the path that are hard to overcome on our own but that an experienced teacher can identify and help to remove. This is an important point that should not be forgotten.

Our human lives are precious. We have intact bodies and minds with complete potential. We may have met teachers and received teachings, and we have lives in which we enjoy the freedom to follow the spiritual path. We know practice is essential to the spiritual journey as well as to our aspiration to help others. We also know life passes quickly and death is certain, yet in our busy lives we find it difficult to practice as much as we wish we could. Perhaps we meditate for an hour or two each day, but that leaves the other twenty-two hours in which to be distracted and tossed about on the waves of *samsara*. But there is always time for sleep. The third of our lives spent sleeping can be a time for practice.

The main theme of this book is that through practice we can cultivate greater awareness during every moment of life. If we do, freedom and flexibility continually increase as we are less governed by habitual preoccupations and distractions. We develop a stable and vivid presence that allows us to choose positive responses to whatever arises, responses that best benefit others and our own spiritual journey. Eventually we develop a continuity of awareness that allows us to maintain full awareness during dream as well as in waking life. Then we are able to respond to dream phenomena in creative and positive ways and can accomplish various practices in the dream state. When we fully develop this capacity, we find we are living both waking and dreaming life with greater ease, comfort, clarity, and appreciation. We will also be preparing ourselves to attain liberation in the intermediate state (*bardo*) after death.

The teachings provide us with many methods to improve the quality of ordinary life. That is good; this life is important. But the ultimate use of these yogas is to lead us to liberation. To that end, this book supplies the practitioner with a practice manual, a guide to the yogas of the Bön-Buddhist traditions of Tibet that use dream to attain liberation from the delusions of ordinary life and use sleep to wake from the darkness of ignorance. To use the book most effectively, stabilize the mind through the practice of calm abiding (*zhiné*) explained in part three. Begin the foundational practices and spend time with them, integrating them into your life. When you think it's time, begin the primary practices. If possible, it's helpful to make a connection with a qualified teacher.

Take the time needed to obtain results. There is no hurry. We have wandered in the samsara for time without measure. To read another book and then forget it will not change your life. But if we follow these practices to their end, we will wake to our primordial nature, enlightenment itself.

If we cannot remain present during sleep, if we lose ourselves every night, what chance do we have of being aware when death comes? If we enter our dreams and interact with the mind's images as if they are real, we should not expect to be free in the state after death. Look to your experience in dreams to know how you will fare in death. Look to your experience of sleep to discover whether or not you are truly awake.

Receiving the Teachings

The best approach to receiving oral and written spiritual teachings is to "hear, conclude, and experience." If learning is approached in this way, the process of learning is continuous and unceasing. But if it stops at the level of the intellect, it can become a barrier to practice.

As to hearing or receiving the teachings, the good student is like a glue-covered wall; weeds thrown against it stick. A weaker student is like a dry wall; what is tossed against it slides to the floor. When the teachings are received, they should not be lost or wasted. Instead, retain the teachings in the mind and work with them. Teachings not penetrated with understanding are like weeds thrown against the dry wall. They fall to the floor and are forgotten.

Concluding means to fully comprehend what is taught, to come to certainty of the meaning of the teaching and how to apply it in practice. Like bringing light to a dark room; what was hidden becomes clear. It's something we now know rather than something we have merely heard. For example, being told a bowl in a dark room is filled with salt is abstract. We can't see the salt. When a light is turned on, we see it directly; we can look in the bowl and be certain it is filled with salt. The teaching is no longer something we can only repeat; we know it to be true.

By "applying in practice," we mean turning what has been conceptually understood—what has been received, pondered, and made meaningful—into direct experience. This process is analogous to tasting salt. Salt can be seen and talked about, its chemical nature understood and so on, but the direct experience is in tasting it. That experience cannot be grasped intellectually and cannot be conveyed in words. If we try to explain it to someone who has never tasted salt, they will not be able to understand what we have experienced. But when we talk of it to someone who has had the experience, then we both know what is being referred to. It is the same with the teachings.

This is how to apply the teachings: hear or read the teachings, study them enough to become certain of the meaning and then realize the meaning through direct experience.

In Tibet, new leather skins are put in the sun and rubbed with butter to make them softer. The beginning practitioner is like the new skin, tough and hard with narrow views and conceptual rigidity.

The teaching (dharma) is like the butter, rubbed in through practice, and the sun is like direct experience. When both are applied, the practitioner becomes soft and flexible. But butter is also stored in leather bags. When butter is left in a bag for some years, the leather of the bag becomes hard as wood, and no amount of new butter can soften it. Someone who spends many years studying the teachings, intellectualizing a great deal with little experience of practice, is like that hardened leather. The teachings can soften the hard skin of ignorance and conditioning, but when they are stored in the intellect and not rubbed into the practitioner with practice and warmed with direct experience, that person may become rigid and hard in their intellectual understanding. We must be careful not to store up the teachings as only conceptual understanding lest that understanding become a block to wisdom. The teachings are not ideas to be collected but a path to be followed.

PART ONE

The Nature of Dream

CHAPTER 1

Dream and Reality

All of us dream whether we remember dreaming or not. We dream as infants and continue dreaming until we die. Every night we enter an unknown world. We may seem to be our ordinary selves or someone completely different. We meet people we know or don't know, who are living or dead. We fly; encounter nonhuman beings; have blissful experiences; laugh; weep; and we may be frightened, exalted, or inspired. Yet we generally pay these extraordinary experiences little attention. Many Westerners who approach the teachings do so with ideas about dream based in psychological theory; subsequently, when they become more interested in using dream in their spiritual lives, they usually focus on the content and meaning of dreams. Rarely is the nature of dreaming itself investigated. When it is, the investigation leads to the mysterious processes that underlie the whole of our existence, not only our dreaming life.

The first step in dream practice is simple: one must recognize the potential dream holds for the spiritual journey. Normally a dream is thought to be "unreal," as opposed to "real" waking life. But waking life, too, is dreamlike. We spend most of our waking time in the dreams of the moving mind. This is why dream yoga applies to all experience, to the dreams of the night and the dreams of the day.

CHAPTER 2

How Experience Is Shaped

Ignorance

All experience, including dream, is shaped by ignorance. This is a startling statement to make in the West, so first let us understand what is meant by "ignorance" (*ma-rigpa*).

The Tibetan tradition distinguishes two kinds of ignorance: innate ignorance and cultural ignorance. Innate ignorance is the basis of samsara and the defining characteristic of ordinary beings. It is ignorance of our true nature and the true nature of the world, resulting in entanglement with the delusions of the dualistic mind.

Dualism reifies polarities and dichotomies. It divides the seamless unity of experience into this and that, right and wrong, you and me. Based on these conceptual divisions, we develop preferences that manifest as grasping and aversion, the habitual responses to life making up most of what we identify as ourselves. We want this, not that; believe in this, not that; respect this and disdain that. We want pleasure, comfort, wealth, respect, and love; and we try to escape pain, poverty, shame, and discomfort. We want an experience different from the one we are having, or we want to hold on to an experience and avoid the inevitable changes that will lead to its cessation.

Beliefs, preferences, and aversions become institutionalized in a culture and codified in value systems. For example, in India, Hindus believe it is wrong to eat cows but fine to eat pigs. Muslims believe it is appropriate to eat beef but they are prohibited from eating pork. Tibetans eat both. Who is right? The Hindu thinks the Hindus are right, the Muslim thinks the Muslims are right, the Tibetan thinks the Tibetans are right. These differences arise from collective biases and beliefs embedded in the culture, not from fundamental wisdom.

Cultural ignorance is developed and preserved in traditions. As we grow up and learn about the world, we naturally become attached to various beliefs, to a political party, a medical system, a religion, and opinions about how things are and should be. Much of our education reinforces the habit of seeing the world through a certain lens, as does the news we read and the media we consume. We grow attached to even small things—a brand of clothing, sitting in a certain chair, a genre of music—and often think our preferences are "better." On a grand scale, we develop competing religions, governments, philosophies, and psychologies.

None of this would be a problem if we accepted differences, but too often we don't. Sports fans may erupt in anger with each other for supporting one team rather than another. Adherents of one political party become furious with a different political party. Religions go to war with each other over differences of belief; even different factions of the same religion have warred against one another.

Ignorance is not "bad." It's the way things are. Ignorance is simply an obscuration of consciousness: condemning it is like being angry at clouds for blocking the sun. Preferences and aversions lead to war but also to humanitarian acts; to weapons and helpful technologies, to medicines and arts, and to greed and corruption; to cruelty and kindness. As long as we are unenlightened, we participate in this. And that is okay. In Tibetan there is a saying: "When in the body of a donkey, enjoy the taste of grass." Appreciate and value this life because it is the life you are living. It is full of beauty and possibilities, including the possibility of enlightenment.

Actions and Results: Karma and Karmic Traces

Suffering is rooted in our minds. We blame our unhappiness on our situation and believe we would be happy if we could change our circumstances. But the situation in which we find ourselves is only the secondary cause of our suffering. The primary cause is innate ignorance and the resulting desire for things to be other than they are. We carry the root of suffering, ignorance of our true nature, with us wherever we go.

Maybe we decide to escape the stresses of the city by moving to the seacoast or the mountains. Or we may leave the isolation and difficulties of the country for the excitement of the city. The change can be good because the secondary causes are altered, and contentment may be found. But only for a while. The root of our discontent moves with us to our new home; from it grow new dissatisfactions. Soon we are again caught up in the turmoil of hope and fear.

Or we may think more money, a better partner, or a better body or job will make us happy. But if we are honest with ourselves, we know this won't last. The rich aren't free from suffering, a new partner will dissatisfy us in some way, the body will age, the new job will grow less interesting. When we think the solution to unhappiness will be found in the external world, we look in the wrong place. We find happiness, but it passes. Not only does this constant dissatisfaction prevent us from finding contentment and happiness in our daily lives but it distracts us from the spiritual path. Tossed this way and that by our always changing desires, we are governed by our karma and continually plant the seeds of future karmic harvests.

Karma means "action" in Sanskrit. *Karmic traces* are the results of actions that remain in the mental consciousness, influencing our future. We can partially understand karmic traces if we think of them as tendencies in the unconscious. They are inclinations, patterns of internal and external behavior, ingrained reactions, habitual conceptualizations. They dictate our characteristic emotional habits and intellectual rigidities. They condition every reaction we normally have to every element of experience.

Here is an example of karmic traces on a gross level, though the same dynamic is at work in even the subtlest experience. A man grows up in a home in which there is a lot of fighting. Thirty or forty years after leaving home, he walks down a street, passing a house in which people are arguing loudly. That night he has a dream in which he is fighting with his spouse or partner. When he wakes in the morning, he feels aggrieved and withdrawn. This is noticed by his partner who reacts to the mood, which irritates him further.

When the man was young, he reacted to the fighting in his home with fear, anger, or hurt. He felt aversion toward the fighting, a normal response, and this aversion left traces in his mind. Decades later he passes a house and hears fighting; this is the secondary condition needed to stimulate the old karmic trace, which manifests in a dream that night, though it could instead manifest as a mood, behavior, or chain of thoughts and memories.

In the dream, the man reacts to his dream partner's provocation with feelings of anger and hurt. This reaction is governed by the karmic traces collected in his mental consciousness as a child and probably reinforced many times since. When the dream partner— who is wholly a projection of the man's mind—provokes him, his reaction is aversion. The aversion he feels in the dream is a new action, creating a new trace and reinforcing the old pattern. When he wakes, he is stuck in negative emotions, the fruit of prior karmas. He feels estranged and withdrawn from his real partner. To complicate matters further, the partner reacts from their own habitual tendencies, perhaps becoming irritated, withdrawn, apologetic, or subservient, and the man reacts negatively.

Any reaction to any situation—external or internal, waking or dreaming—if conditioned by grasping or aversion, leaves a trace. As karma dictates reactions, the reactions reinforce the karmic tendencies, which further dictate reactions, and so on. This is how karma leads to more karma. It is the wheel of samsara, the ceaseless cycle of conditioned action and reaction.

Obscurations of Consciousness

Karmic traces are like seeds. An apple seed needs the right combination of moisture, light, nutrients, and temperature to sprout and grow. Karmic seeds similarly need the right situation to manifest. The elements supporting the manifestation of the karma are known as secondary causes and conditions and can be an environment, in incident, a person, thoughts, or memories. The seeds are stored in the base consciousness of the individual, in the *kunzhi namshe*.

The common metaphor for the kunzhi namshe is of a storehouse or repository, but it is not a thing or place. It is equivalent to all obscurations of consciousness; when there are no obscurations of consciousness, there is no kunzhi namshe. Until then, it underlies dualistic experience, manifesting as habitual reactions, inclinations, and identities.

When death comes and the body deteriorates, the kunzhi namshe does not. The karmic traces continue in the mental continuum until they are purified. When they are completely gone, there is no longer a kunzhi namshe, and the individual is a buddha.

Positive and Negative Karma

It's helpful to think of karma as cause and effect; actions and reactions have consequences. Popularly, karma is thought of as reward or punishment: you do wrong, bad things happen to you; do right, and good things happen. If you suffer misfortune, it's because of something you did previously; good fortune arrives because of positive actions you took in the past. But karma is not a cosmic tally that is balanced through positive and negative events in your life. Karma is conditioning arising from your repeated reactions to experience. Once we understand that each karmic trace is a seed for further karmically governed action, we also understand how to begin to avoid creating negativity and instead create conditions to influence our lives in a positive direction.

Negative Karma

If we react to a situation with negative emotion, the trace left in the mind will influence future experience negatively. For example, if someone is angry with us and we react with anger, we are left with a seed making it slightly more likely for anger to arise in us again, and it becomes more likely that we will encounter the secondary situations that allow our habitual anger to arise. This is easy to see if we have a great deal of anger in our lives or if we know someone who does. Angry people continually encounter situations that seem to justify their anger, while people with less anger do not. The external situations may be similar, but the different karmic inclinations create different subjective worlds.

If an emotion is expressed impulsively, it can generate strong results and reactions. Anger can lead to a fight or some kind of destruction. People can be harmed physically or emotionally. This is not true of just anger. If envy is strong, it can create great stress for the person who suffers it; it can alienate that person from others, and so on. It is not difficult to see how this leads to negative traces that influence the future negatively.

If we suppress emotion, there is still a negative trace. Suppression is a manifestation of aversion. We tighten inside ourselves, putting something behind a door and locking it, forcing part of our experience into the dark where it waits until the appropriate secondary cause calls it out. This may manifest in many ways. For example, if we suppress our jealousy of others, it may eventually manifest in an emotional outburst or lead us to harshly judge others of whom we are secretly jealous, even if we deny this jealousy to ourselves. Mental judgment is also an action, based on aversion, that creates negative karmic seeds.

Positive Karma

Instead of reacting to situations blindly, we can take a moment to stop and communicate with ourselves. In that space, we can choose to generate the antidote to the negative emotion rather than act it out. If someone is angry with us and our own anger arises, the antidote is compassion. Inducing it may feel forced and inauthentic at first, but if we realize the person irritating us is being controlled by their own conditioning, we can feel compassion, maybe even a connection to the person, and start to let go of our negative reactions. As we do, we begin to shape our future positively.

This new response is still based on desire—in this case, for virtue, peace, or spiritual growth—and produces a karmic trace, a positive one. We have planted a seed of compassion. The next time we encounter anger, we are a little more likely to respond with compassion, which is much more comfortable and spacious than the narrowness of self-protective anger. In this way, the practice of virtue cumulatively retrains our response to the world and we find ourselves, for instance, encountering less and less anger both internally and externally. If we continue in this practice, we begin to see fewer people who seem to deserve our condemnation or anger and more people grappling with karmic conditioning. Compassion eventually arises spontaneously and without effort.

Using the understanding of karma, we can retrain our minds to use all experience, even the most private and fleeting daydreams, to support spiritual practice.

Liberating Emotions

The best response to negative emotion is to allow it to self-liberate by remaining in clear, nonreactive awareness, free of grasping and aversion. If we can do this, the emotion passes through us like a bird flying through space; no trace of its passage remains. The emotion arises and spontaneously dissolves in the clear space of awareness.

In this case, the karmic seed is manifesting—as emotion or thought or bodily sensation or an impulse toward particular behaviors—but because we do not react with grasping or aversion, no seed of future karma is generated. Every time jealously, for example, is allowed to arise and dissolve in awareness without our becoming caught by it or trying to repress it, the strength of the karmic tendency toward envy weakens. There is no new action to reinforce it. Liberating emotion in this way cuts karma at its root, burning the karmic seeds before they have an opportunity to grow into trouble in our lives.

You may ask why it is better to liberate emotion rather than generate positive karma. All karmic traces act to constrain us, to restrict us to particular identities. The goal of the path is complete liberation from all conditioning. This does not mean that once one is liberated positive traits such as compassion are not present. They are. But when no longer driven by karmic tendencies, we see our situation clearly and respond spontaneously and appropriately rather than being pushed in one direction or pulled in another. Relative compassion arising from positive karmic tendencies is very good. Better is the absolute compassion arising effortlessly in the individual liberated from karmic conditioning. It is more spacious and inclusive, more effective, and free of delusion.

Allowing emotion to self-liberate is the best response, but it is difficult to accomplish before practice is developed and stable. However our practice is now, all of us can determine to stop for a moment when emotion arises, check in with ourselves, and choose to act as skillfully as possible. We can all learn to blunt the force of impulse, of karmic habits. We can remind ourselves that the emotion we are experiencing is simply a conditioned response, that it doesn't help us or the other person. We relax our identification with the emotion or point of view and let go of our defensiveness. As the tension loosens, we become more spacious internally and more able to respond positively, planting seeds of positive karma. Again, it is important to do this without repressing emotion. We should relax as we generate compassion, not tightly suppress anger in the body while trying to think good thoughts.

The spiritual journey is not meant to benefit only the far future or our next life. As we practice training ourselves to react more positively to situations, we change our karmic traces and develop qualities that effect positive changes in the lives we are leading right now. As we see more clearly that every experience, however small and private, has a result, we can use this to change our lives and our dreams.

Karmic Traces and Dream

All samsaric experience is shaped by karmic traces. Moods, thoughts, emotions, mental images, perceptions, instinctive reactions, "common sense," and even our sense of identity are governed by the workings of karma. For example, you may wake up feeling down. You have breakfast, everything seems to be okay but there is a sense of unhappiness that cannot be accounted for. We say in this case that some karma is ripening. The causes and conditions have come together in such a way that depression manifests. There may be a hundred reasons for this depression to occur on this particular morning, and it may manifest in a myriad of ways. It may also manifest during the night as a dream.

During the day, consciousness illuminates the senses and we experience the world, weaving sensory and psychic experiences into the meaningful whole of our lives. At night, consciousness withdraws from the senses and resides in the base. If we have developed a strong practice of presence with much experience of the nature of mind, we will rest in lucid awareness. But for most of us, consciousness illuminates the obscurations and these manifest as a dream.

Karmic traces are like photos, videos, and memories we collect. Any experience we react to with desire or aversion is recorded and stored in the kunzhi namshe. Depending on the secondary conditions encountered during the day, certain traces are stimulated. In the darkroom of our sleep, the mind weaves these influences into the narrative of the dream, as narrative is how the mind makes meaning. This is a dream, constructed from memories, conditioned tendencies and habitual identities. While we are in the dream, it is as real to us as waking life.

Although the dynamics are easier to understand in dream, where they are free of the limitations of the physical world and the rational consciousness, the same dream-making process continues in waking life. We project this activity of the mind onto the world and think, as we do in the dreams of night, that the objects we encounter and their qualities exist independently of our minds. They don't.

As described earlier, in dream yoga this understanding of karma is used to train the mind to react differently to experience, resulting in new karmic traces. As we make progress in the practice, dreams more conducive to spiritual practice are generated. It is not about force, about consciousness acting to oppress the unconscious.

Dream yoga relies instead on increased awareness and insight to enable us to make positive choices that lead to increased lucidity in dream and waking. We change the underlying traces driving the creation of dreams of night and day.

In dream we can burn the seeds of future karma just as we can in waking life. If we abide in nonreactive awareness during a dream, we can allow karmic traces to self-liberate as they arise. If this is not possible for us yet, we can still develop tendencies to choose spiritually positive behavior in our dreams until we go beyond preferences and dualism altogether.

The Six Realms of Cyclic Existence

In Bön and Buddhist cosmology, all deluded beings exist in one of six realms (loka). These are the realms of gods, demigods, humans, animals, hungry ghosts, and hell beings. Fundamentally, the realms are six dimensions of consciousness, six dimensions of possible experience. They manifest in us when we experience the six negative emotions: anger, greed, ignorance, jealousy, pride, and pleasurable distraction. (Pleasurable distraction is the emotional state when the other five emotions are harmoniously balanced.) According to the teaching, the six realms are not only categories of emotional experience; they are actual realms into which beings are born, just as we were born into the human realm and a lion was born into the animal realm.

Each realm can be thought of as a continuum of experience. The hell realm, for instance, ranges from individuals' internal emotional experience of anger and hatred and behaviors rooted in those emotions; to social manifestations like prejudices, intolerance, and oppression; and as an actual realm in which beings exist. A name for the entirety of this dimension of experience, from individual emotion to the actual realm, is "hell."

Like dreams, the realms are manifestations of karmic traces, but in the instance of the realms, the karmic traces are collective rather than individual. Because the karma is collective, the beings in each realm share similar experiences in a consensual world, as we share similar experiences with other humans. Collective karma creates bodies and senses and mental capacities, allowing individuals to participate in shared potentials and categories of experience while making other kinds of experience impossible. Dogs, for example, can collectively hear sounds humans cannot, and humans experience language in a way dogs cannot.

The realms appear to be distinct and solid, as our world seems to us, but they are actually dreamy and insubstantial. They interpenetrate one another; we are connected to each and carry the seeds of rebirth into the other realms with us. When we experience different emotions, we participate in some of the characteristic qualities and suffering predominant in other realms. When we are caught up in self-centered pride or angry envy, for example, we experience something of the characteristic quality of experience of the demigod realm.

Some individuals have a predominance of one dimension in their makeup: more animal, more hungry ghost, more god nature, or more demigod. It stands out as a dominant trait. We may know people who seem to be trapped in the hungry ghost realm: they can never get enough, are always hungry for more—more from friends, from their environment, from their lives—but can never be satisfied. Or we know someone who seems like a hell being: angry, violent, raging, in turmoil. More commonly, people have aspects of all the dimensions in their individual makeup.

As these dimensions of consciousness manifest in emotions, it becomes apparent how universal they are. For example, every culture knows anger. The appearance of anger may vary because emotional expression is a means of communication determined by both biology and culture, and culture provides the variable. But the feeling of anger is the same everywhere. In Bön-Buddhism, this universality is explained by and correlated with the realms.

The six negative emotions are not meant to constitute an exhaustive list of emotions. For example, grief and anxiety are not mentioned very much but both can be experienced in any of the realms, as can anger or jealousy or love. We have the seeds of all realms and all experiences in us right now.

The six qualities of consciousness are called paths because they lead somewhere: they take us to the places of our birth and into different realms of experience in life. When a being identifies with or is ensnared in certain kinds of experience, there are results. This works positively and negatively. For example, we believe that to be born as a human, we must have been involved in moral disciplines in previous lifetimes. Even in popular culture this is expressed in the observation that it is not until love and concern for others matures that a person is considered "fully human."

If we live a life characterized by hatred and anger, we experience a different result: we are reborn in hell. This happens physically—a being may be born in the hell realm—as well as psychologically in this life.

This does not mean humans necessarily try to avoid the experiences we are calling negative. We often entertain ourselves by watching movies, playing video games, and reading books featuring conflict, hatred, murder, revenge, and war. "War is hell," we say, yet many of us are drawn to war.

Our bias toward one or another of these dimensions is also shaped by culture. For instance, in a society in which the angry warrior is considered heroic, we may be led in that direction, whereas if success at all costs is the ideal, greed and envy may be pervasive. This is an example of cultural ignorance.

The realms may sound fanciful to people in the West. You needn't believe they are "real" to recognize the manifestation of the six realms in experience.

We may experience the happiness of the god realm while on vacation or on a walk with friends; the ache of greed when obsessed with something we feel we must have; the shame of wounded pride; the pangs of jealousy; the hellishness of bitterness and hatred; the dullness and confusion of ignorance. We move from the experience of one realm to another easily and frequently.

We have the experience of being in a happy mood, connected to the god realm—the sun is out, people appear beautiful, we feel good about life and ourselves. Then we receive bad news, or a friend says something that hurts us. Suddenly our experience changes. There's no reason to smile, we don't see the beauty we did minutes ago, we no longer find others attractive, nor do we enjoy ourselves. We have changed dimensions of experience, and our world changed with us.

During our dreaming lives, too, we experience the six realms. Just as they determine the quality of experience during the day, they shape the feeling and content of dreams.

The table below gives a brief description of the six realms. Traditionally, the realms are presented as descriptions of places and the beings who inhabit those places. The hells, for example, are eighteen in number, but here we are focused on the experiences of the realms in this life. We connect to each dimension of experience energetically through an energy center (chakra) in the body, the locations of which are listed in the table. The chakras are important in many different practices and play a role in dream yoga.

Realm	Primary Emotion	Chakra
God (*devas*)	Pleasurable distraction	Crown
Demigod (*asuras*)	Envy/Pride	Throat
Human	Jealousy	Heart
Animal	Ignorance	Navel
Hungry ghost (*pretas*)	Greed	Sexual organs
Hell	Hatred/Anger	Soles of the feet

Hell Realm

Anger is the seed emotion of the hell realm. When the karmic traces of anger manifest, there are many possible expressions: aversion, tension, resentment, criticism, argument, and violence. Much of the destruction of wars is caused by anger, and many people die every day as a result of it. Yet anger never resolves any problem.

When it overcomes us, we lose control and self-awareness. When we are trapped in hatred, violence, and anger, we are participating in the hell realm.

The energetic center of anger is in the soles of the feet. The antidote for anger is unconditioned love, which arises from the unconditioned nature of mind.

Traditionally, the hells are said to be composed of nine hot hells and nine cold hells. The beings who live there suffer immeasurably, being tortured to death and instantly returning to life time after time.

Hungry Ghost Realm

Greed is the seed emotion of the hungry ghost (preta) realm. Greed arises as a feeling of excessive need that cannot be fulfilled. The attempt to satisfy greed is like drinking salty water when we are thirsty. When lost in greed, we look outward rather than inward for satisfaction, never finding enough to fill the emptiness we wish to escape. The real hunger we feel is for knowledge of our true nature.

Greed is associated with sexual desire; its energetic center in the body is the chakra behind the genitals. Generosity, the open giving of what others need, is the remedy for greed.

The pretas are traditionally represented as beings with huge, hungry bellies and tiny mouths and throats. Some inhabit parched lands where there is not even a mention of water for hundreds of years. Others may find food and drink, yet if they swallow even a little through their tiny mouths, the food bursts into flame in their stomachs and causes great pain. There are many kinds of suffering for pretas, but all result from greed and opposing the generosity of others.

Animal Realm

Ignorance is the seed of the animal realm. It is experienced as a feeling of being lost, dull, uncertain, or unaware. Many people experience a darkness and sadness rooted in this ignorance; they feel a need but do not know what they want or what to do to satisfy themselves. In the West, people are often considered happy if they are continually busy, but we can be lost in ignorance in the midst of our busyness when we do not know our true nature.

The chakra associated with ignorance is in the center of the body at the level of the navel. The wisdom found when we turn inward and come to know our true nature is the antidote to ignorance.

Beings in the animal realm are dominated by the darkness of ignorance. Many animals live in fear because of the constant threat from other animals and humans. Even large animals are tormented by insects burrowing into their skin and living on their flesh. Domesticated animals are milked, loaded down, castrated, pierced through the nose, and ridden, with no hope of escape. Animals feel pain and pleasure but are dominated by the ignorance preventing them from looking beneath the circumstances of their lives to find their true nature.

Human Realm

Jealousy is the root emotion of the human realm. When possessed by jealousy, we want to hold on to what we have and draw to ourselves what others have: an idea, a possession, a relationship, success, respect, accomplishments. We see the source of happiness as something external to us, which leads to greater attachment to the object of our desire.

Jealousy is related to the heart center in the body. The antidote to jealousy is great openness of the heart, the openness arising when we connect to our true nature.

It is easy for us to observe the suffering of our own realm. We experience birth, sickness, old age, and death. We are plagued by loss due to constant change. When we attain the object of our desire, we struggle to keep it, but its eventual loss is certain. Rather than rejoicing in the happiness of others, we often fall prey to envy and jealousy. Even though human birth is considered the greatest of good fortune because humans have the chance to hear and practice the teachings, only a tiny minority of us ever find our way to, and avail ourselves of, this great opportunity.

Demigod Realm

Pride is the principal affliction of the demigods (asuras). Pride is a feeling connected to accomplishment and is often territorial. One cause of war is the pride of individuals and nations that believe they have the solution to other people's problems. There is a hidden aspect of pride that manifests when we believe ourselves worse than others, a negative self-centeredness separating us from others.

Pride is associated with the chakra in the throat. Pride is often manifested in wrathful action. Its antidote is the great peace and humility arising as we rest in our true nature.

The asuras enjoy pleasure and abundance but tend toward envy and wrath. They continually fight with one another, but their greatest suffering occurs when they declare war on the gods, who enjoy even greater abundance than the demigods. The gods are more powerful than asuras and very difficult to kill. They always win the wars, and asuras suffer the emotional devastation of wounded pride and envy in which they feel diminished and that, in turn, drives them into futile wars again and again.

God Realm

Pleasurable distraction is the seed of the god (deva) realm. In the god realm, the five negative emotions are equally present, balanced like five harmonious voices in a chorus. The gods are lost in a heady sense of lazy joy and self-centered pleasure. They enjoy great wealth and comfort during lives lasting as long as an eon. All needs seem to be fulfilled and all desires sated. Just as is true for some individuals and societies, the gods become trapped in pleasure and the pursuit of pleasure. They have no sense of the reality beneath their experience. Lost in meaningless diversions and pleasures, they are too distracted to follow the path to liberation.

But the situation ultimately changes as the karmic causes for existence in the god realm are exhausted. As death finally approaches, the dying god is abandoned by friends and companions unable to face the proof of their own mortality. The previously perfect body ages and deteriorates. The period of happiness is over. With divine eyes the god sees the conditions of the realm of suffering into which they are fated to be reborn. Even before death, the suffering of the coming life begins.

The god realm is associated with the chakra at the crown of the head. The antidote to the selfish joy of the gods is the encompassing compassion that arises spontaneously through awareness of the reality underlying self and world.

Why "Negative" Emotion?

Many people in the West are uncomfortable when they hear emotions labeled as negative. It is not that emotions in themselves are negative. All emotions aid in survival and are necessary for the full range of human experience, including those of attachment, anger, pride, jealousy, and so on. Without the emotions, we would not live fully.

However, emotions are negative insofar as we become ensnared in them and lose touch with the deeper aspects of ourselves. More exactly, it is our reactions to the emotions that become negative, the grasping or aversion, as they lead to a constriction of consciousness and identity. This sows the seeds of future negative conditions, trapping us in realms of suffering in this and subsequent lives. This is negative when compared to a more expansive identity, particularly when compared to liberation from all contrived and constricted identities. This is why it is helpful to think of the realms not just as emotional states but as six dimensions of consciousness and experience.

If we understand the empty nature of reality, it is easier to let go of grasping and therefore there is no grosser form of the emotion. In absolute reality, there is no separate entity to serve as the target of our anger or the object of any emotion. There is no reason to get angry at all. We create the story, the projections, and the anger at the same time.

Often in the West, the understanding of emotions is used in psychology to improve people's lives in samsara. That is good. However, the Tibetan system has a different goal. The understanding of emotions is used to free ourselves of the constrictions and erroneous views we are bound to through emotional attachment. Emotions are negative to the extent that we cling to them or flee from them.

CHAPTER 3

The Energy Body

All experience has an energetic basis. This vital energy is called *lung* in Tibetan, but it is better known in the West by its Sanskrit name, *prana*. The underlying structure of any experience is a combination of various conditions and causes. If we are able to understand why and how an experience is occurring, and to recognize its mental, physical, and energetic dynamics, then we can reproduce those experiences or alter them. This allows us to generate experiences that support spiritual practice and avoid those that are detrimental.

Channels and Prana

In daily life, we take different bodily positions without thinking of their effects. When we want to relax and talk with friends, we go to a room with comfortable chairs or sofas. This increases the experience of calm and relaxation and is conducive to easy conversation. When we are active in business discussions, we go to an office where the chairs hold us more erect and less relaxed. This is more supportive of business and creative endeavors. If we want to rest in silence, we might go to the porch and sit in still another kind of chair, situated so that we can enjoy the landscape and the flow of air. When we grow tired, we go to the bedroom and take a completely different posture to induce sleep.

Similarly, we assume various postures in different types of meditation to alter the flow of prana in the body by manipulating the channels (*tsa*), which are the conduits of energy in the body, and to open different energetic focal points, the chakras. Doing this changes our experience. This is the basis for the movements of yoga. Consciously guiding the energy in the body allows for an easier and more rapid development of meditation practice than would occur if we relied only on the mind. It also allows us to overcome certain obstacles in practice. Without using the knowledge of prana and its movement in the body, the mind can become mired in its own processes.

Channels, prana, and chakras are involved in death as well as life. Most mystical experience, as well as experiences in the intermediate state after death, result from the opening and closing of energy points. Many books reporting on the phenomena of near-death experiences contain descriptions of various lights and visions people experience as the death process begins. According to the Tibetan tradition, these phenomena have to do with the movement of prana. The channels are associated with different elements; during the dissolution of the elements at death, as the channels deteriorate, the released energy manifests in experience as light and color. The teachings go into great detail about which colored light corresponds to the dissolution of which channel, where it is in the body, and to which emotion it is related.

There is considerable variation in how these lights appear to us at death because they are related to both negative and positive aspects of consciousness. The average person experiences emotions at death, and the dominant emotion determines which lights and colors manifest. Often there is, at first, only an experience of colored lights in which one color is primary, but it may also be the case that a few colors are predominant, or there is a combination of many colors. The light then begins to form images, as it does in dreams: houses, castles, mandalas, people, deities, almost anything. When we are dying, we may relate to these visions as either real entities, in which case we are governed by our reactions to them in moving toward our next birth, or as meditative experiences, which allows us the opportunity of liberation, or at least the possibility of consciously influencing our next birth in a positive direction.

Channels (*Tsa*)

There are different kinds of channels in the body. We know of the grosser channels through the medical study of anatomy, from which we learn about blood vessels, the circulation of lymph, the network of nerves, and so on. There are also conduits for the more substantive forms of prana, such as those recognized in acupuncture. In dream yoga we are concerned with a subtler psychic energy underlying both wisdom and negative emotion. The channels carrying this subtle energy cannot be located in the physical dimension, but we can become aware of them.

There are three root channels. Six major chakras are centered in the central channel. From the six chakras, 360 branch channels spread throughout the body. The root channels comprise the white right channel, the red left channel, and the blue central channel.

The central channel begins at the perineum and rises up in front of the spine. It is the diameter of a cane, widening slightly from the heart area to the crown of the head.

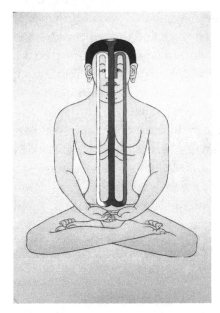

The three primary channels as used in the practices in this book. The side channels go all the way up to the underside of the skull before curving down.

The two side channels, each the diameter of a pencil, form a junction with the central channel four finger widths below the navel. They rise through the center of the body on either side and parallel to the central channel. When they reach the underside of the skull at the crown, instead of exiting through the crown as the central channel does, they follow the curve under the skull, continue down behind the eyes and exit at their respective nostrils.

Contradictions

As you read through this and other books, you'll come across conflicting descriptions of the qualities associated with channels and chakras. For instance, in a later section of this book, the central channel is associated with ignorance. Here, it is associated with nondual awareness. The central channel connects to both: it supports nondual awareness, and that awareness may be obscured by the root poison of ignorance.

There are variations in the descriptions of the white and red channels too. In the first edition of this book, the white and red channels were mirrored in men and women. For women, the white channel was on the left side of the body, and the red channel was on the right. For men, it was the opposite: the white channel on the right side of the body, the red channel on the left. In this edition, they are the same: for both women and men, the white channel is on the right, and the red channel is on the left.

These contradictions are found in different texts, when comparing different traditions, and from one teacher to another. For this edition of the book, I asked a number of lamas I know, both Bön and Nyingma teachers, and found they were split depending on their history, on their tradition, and which texts they used. Some taught the side channels are the same for men and women; some taught they mirror one another.

I asked my root teacher, H. E. Yongdzin Rinpoche, what he recommended. He said to teach that the channels are the same for men and women, so that is how it is taught in this book.

The differences are related to different aspects of the energetic body, to different qualities of the prana depending on mind states, and the different uses of the energy body in the context of different practices. The qualities assigned to different areas of the energy body, the colors and shapes, are symbols that help us focus on qualities of the mind and body. But the symbols in themselves are not real. The channels do not have color, the sizes are not exact. The symbols are only meant to bring your mind, your attention, to the right areas of the body and to qualities to be developed in practice. So don't be confused when you come across these contradictions; just let go and practice as described in the particular teaching.

Here, the blue channel is understood to be the channel of nonduality. It is in this central channel in which the energy of primordial awareness (*rigpa*) moves. Dream practice ultimately brings the consciousness and the prana into the central channel where it abides beyond both negative and positive experience. When this occurs, the practitioner realizes the unity of all apparent dualities. Generally, when people have mystical experiences, great experiences of bliss or emptiness or clarity or rigpa, they are energetically based in the central channel.

Prana (*Lung*)

Dreaming is a dynamic process. The content in dream is fluid: beings move and talk, sounds vibrate, sensation is vivid. The content of a dream is formed by the mind, but the basis of the vitality and animation of the dream is the prana. The literal translation of the Tibetan word for prana, *lung*, is "wind," but it is more descriptive to call it the vital wind force.

Prana is the foundational energy of all experience, of all life. In the East, people practice yoga positions and various breathing exercises to strengthen and refine the vital wind force in order to balance the body and the mind. Some of the ancient Tibetan esoteric teachings describe two different kinds of prana: karmic prana and wisdom prana.

Karmic Prana

When the karmic traces are activated by the appropriate second-ary causes, karmic prana energizes them, allowing them to have an effect in the mind and body, in waking and in dreams. Karmic prana is the vitality of the negative and positive energies in both side channels.

When the mind is unstable, distracted, or unfocused, karmic prana moves. This means, for example, when an emotion arises and the mind is not stable, the karmic prana carries the mind wherever it will. Our attention moves here and there, pushed and pulled by aversion and desire.

Developing mental stability is necessary on the spiritual path to make the mind strong, present, and focused. Then, even when the forces of negative emotions arise, we are not distracted and lost.

Some Tibetan yoga texts describe three kinds of karmic prana: soft prana, rough prana, and neutral prana. Soft prana refers to virtuous wisdom prana, which moves through the red wisdom chan-nel. Rough prana refers to the prana of negative emotion, which moves through the white channel. In this classification, both virtu-ous wisdom prana and emotional prana are karmic prana.

Neutral prana is, as its name suggests, neither virtuous nor non-virtuous, but it is still karmic prana. It pervades the body and is nei-ther negative or positive. Experience of the neutral prana is helpful as a bridge to the experience of wisdom prana.

Wisdom Prana

Wisdom prana (ye lung) is not karmic prana. It is not to be confused with the virtuous wisdom karma described in the last section, which underlies virtuous actions. The wisdom prana here is the energy of nondual experience. It moves through the central channel.

In the first moment of any experience, before a reaction occurs, there is only pure perception. The prana involved in this pure experiencing is the primordial wisdom prana, the energy underlying experience prior to or free of grasping or aversion. This pure experience does not leave a trace and is not the cause of dreams. The wisdom prana is the energy of unconditioned awareness. This moment is very brief, a flash of pure experience of which we are usually unaware. It is our reaction to this moment, our grasping and aversion, that we think of as our experience. Paying attention to the moment of perception before it is conceptualized, and extending the moment, begins to introduce us to pure awareness.

The Tibetan Buddhist teacher Longchenpa says in one text that there are 21,600 movements of prana during a single day. Whether literal or not, the statement indicates the enormous activity of prana and thought occurring each day.

Balancing the Prana

This is a simple practice one can do to balance the prana.

Inhale through both nostrils with a slow, full breath. Imagine inhaling blissful wisdom prana, drawing the breath down to the junction with the central channel. Hold the breath gently and briefly in the relaxed belly, or in any part of the body where there is tension. Feel neutral prana pervade the body. Let body and mind ease and relax.

When ready, exhale fully through both nostrils. Feel all stress and negative rough, emotional prana flow out of the body. At the end of the exhalation, let go into relaxation and rest in the peaceful mind. At any time during the day, you can take a few minutes for this breath. Even three breaths will change your experience positively. Repeating this again and again will balance your energy.

Prana and Mind

All dreams are related to one or more of the six realms. The energetic connection between the mind and the realm is made through specific locations in the body. How can this be? We say that consciousness is beyond shape, color, time, or touch, so how can it be connected to place? The fundamental mind is beyond any such distinctions, but the qualities that arise in consciousness are influenced by the phenomena of experience.

We can look into this question for ourselves. Go somewhere peaceful—a beautiful temple filled with gentle singing and the smell of incense, or the green pool below a small waterfall. When we enter such a place, it's as if a blessing is received. The quality of experience is affected because the physical environment affects the state of consciousness. This is also true for negative influences. When visiting a location that has been the site of atrocities, we become uneasy; we say the place has "bad energy."

The same is true internally, inside our bodies. What do we mean when we talk about bringing the mind to a chakra—to the heart chakra, for example? What does it mean for the mind to be somewhere? Mind cannot be localized or contained in a small area. When we "put" the mind somewhere, we are placing our attention. We are creating images in the mind or directing attention to a sense object. When we focus the mind on something, the object of focus affects the quality of consciousness, and there are correlated changes in the body.

This principle underlies healing practices that make use of mental imagery. Visualization leads to changes in our bodies. Western research is demonstrating the truth of this statement as Western medicine uses the power of visualization for relaxation, relief of stress, overcoming trauma, pain control, and even serious illnesses such as cancer. The Bön tradition of healing often uses visualization of the elements: fire, water, and wind. Rather than addressing symptoms of the disease, the follower of Bön generally attempts to purify the underlying conditioning of the mind, the energetic system, and the negative emotions and karmic traces believed to create susceptibility to disease.

For example, we may visualize intense fire in response to an illness. We visualize red triangular shapes and try to imaginatively experience heat—as powerful as that rising from a volcano—moving through our bodies like waves of flame. We may do a particular breathing exercise to generate even more heat. In this way, we use the mind and its images to affect the body, the emotions, and the energy. And there is a result. As Western medicine may use radiation therapy to attempt to burn cancer cells, we use internal fire to burn up karmic traces. For the practice to be effective, the intention must be clear. It is not a simple mechanical process but one using the understanding of karma, mind, and prana to aid healing. Of course, it is good to avail ourselves of Western medicine when possible. We use whatever is beneficial.

Chakras

In dream practice, we direct our attention to different areas in the body: the chakras at the throat, brow, and heart and the secret chakra behind the genitals. A chakra is a nexus of energetic connections. Channels of energy meet at particular locations in the body; the junctions of the channels form the energetic patterns that are chakras. Major chakras are sites where many channels join. Chakras are not really like the pictures drawn of them, of lotuses that open and close, that have a certain number of petals and are a certain color. Such images are only symbolic supports for the mind, maps we use to help focus the attention on the patterns of energy existing at the sites of the chakras.

The chakras were initially discovered through practice, through the realizations of different practitioners. When these practitioners developed experiences of the chakras, there was no language to describe their discoveries to those who had not had the same experience. Images were created to be used as visual metaphors. The various images of the lotus, for instance, suggested that the energy around a chakra expanded and contracted like the opening and closing of a flower; one chakra felt different from another, and these differences were represented by different colors; experiences of varying concentrations and complexities of energy in the different chakras were represented by different numbers of petals. These visual metaphors became a language used to articulate the experiences of the energy centers in the body. When a new practitioner visualizes the right number of petals at the right spot in the body with the right color, then the power of the mind affects that particular energetic point and is influenced by that point. When this occurs, we say mind and prana are unified in the chakra.

Blind Horse, Lame Rider

At night, when we go to sleep, we generally do so with little sense of what is happening. We just feel tired, shut our eyes, and drift away. We may have an idea about sleep—blood in the brain, hormones, circadian rhythms, or something like that—but the change in consciousness as we fall asleep remains mysterious.

The Tibetan tradition explains the process of falling asleep using metaphors. Often prana is compared to a blind horse and the mind to a person unable to walk. Separately they are limited, but together they make a functional unit. When the horse and rider are together, they begin to run, generally with little control over where they go. We know this from our own experience: we can "put" the mind into a chakra by placing attention there, but it is not easy to keep the mind in any one place. The mind is always moving.

As we fall asleep, awareness of the sensory world is lost. The mind is carried here and there on the blind horse of karmic prana until it becomes focused in a particular chakra, where it is influenced by a particular dimension of consciousness. Perhaps you had a disagreement with someone, and that situation (secondary condition) activates a karmic trace, a conditioning associated with the heart chakra, which pulls your mind to that location in the body. The subsequent activity of mind and prana manifests in the particular images and stories of the dream.

The mind is not driven randomly to one chakra or another. It is drawn to the places in the body and the associated situations in life needing attention and healing. In the example, it's as if the heart chakra is calling for help, asking the awareness to attend to it. The disturbing trace will be healed by manifesting in the dream and thereby being exhausted. However, unless the manifestation takes place while the dreamer is centered and aware, the reactions to it will be dictated by habitual karmic tendencies and will create new and similar karmic seeds.

We can think of a computer as an analogy. The chakras are like different folders. Click on the directory "Prana and Mind," and then open the file of the heart chakra. The information in the file—the karmic traces associated with the heart chakra—is displayed on the screen of awareness. This is like the dream manifesting.

Perhaps a situation in the dream then elicits another response, energizing a different emotion. The dream now becomes the secondary cause that allows another karmic trace to manifest. Maybe the mind now travels to the navel center and enters a different realm of experience. The character of the dream changes. You are not jealous now; instead, you are on a street without signs or somewhere very dark. You are lost. You try to go somewhere but can't find your way. You are in the animal realm, the dimension most connected to cognitive ignorance.

Basically, this is how the content of a dream is shaped. The mind and prana are drawn to different chakras in the body. Shaped by the associated karmic traces, experiences arise in the mind as the content of a dream. We can use this understanding to look at our dreams differently, to notice which emotion and realm is connected to a specific dream. It is also helpful to understand that every dream offers an opportunity for healing and spiritual practice.

Ultimately, we wish to stabilize the mind and the prana in the central channel rather than allowing the mind to be drawn to a particular chakra. The central channel is the energetic basis of experiences of rigpa. The practices of dream yoga are meant to bring mind and prana into the central channel. When this occurs, we remain in clear awareness and strong presence. To dream in the central channel is to dream free of influences from the negative emotions. It is a balanced situation that allows dreams of knowledge and clarity to manifest.

CHAPTER 4

Summary: How Dreams Arise

Prior to realization, the individual's true nature is obscured by the root ignorance that gives rise to the conceptual mind. Ensnared in dualistic vision, the conceptual mind divides the seamless unity of experience into conceptual entities and then relates to these mental projections as if they inherently exist as separate beings and things. This misunderstanding divides experience into self and other, and from the identification with only one aspect of experience—the self—preferences develop. This results in the arising of aversion and desire, which become the basis for both physical and mental actions. These actions (karmas) leave traces, conditioning the mind and resulting in more grasping and aversion, which lead to new karmic traces, and so on. This is the self-perpetuating cycle of karma.

During sleep, the mind is withdrawn from the sensory world. Karmic traces currently stimulated by the secondary causes necessary for their manifestation have a force or energy that is the karmic prana. Like the horse and rider in the analogy, the mind "rides" the karmic prana to the energetic center in the body related to the activated karmic trace. That is, the consciousness becomes focused in a particular chakra and a particular dimension of experience.

In this interplay of mind, energy, and meaning, consciousness illuminates and is affected by the karmic traces. The karmic prana is the energy of the dream, the vital force, while the mind weaves the specific manifestations of the karmic traces—the color, light, emotions, and images—into the narrative that is the dream. This is the process resulting in samsaric dreams.

CHAPTER 5

Images from the *Mother Tantra*

In the Great Perfection (Dzogchen) teachings, the issue is always whether or not we recognize our true nature and understand that all experiences are reflections of our own mind. This is easy to believe about a dream after we wake up, just as the buddhas know, after enlightenment, that the entities and objects of samsara are empty appearances. Understanding how dreams arise makes it easier to see the same processes at work during the day, and easier to understand what is meant by "illusory" and "lacking inherent existence"

There is a Tibetan term, *lhun drub*, that translates as "spontaneous perfection." It means there is no producer producing anything. Everything is just as it is, arising from the base as a spontaneous manifestation of emptiness and clarity. The mirror does not select a face to reflect: its nature is to reflect everything. Clear awareness is like the mirror. When we see everything as a spontaneously arising reflection of mind, including our conventional sense of self, we approach freedom. Without this understanding, the sense of separation is strong and we struggle with illusions. There is no place where the dream breaks until we are awake in undeluded awareness.

The *Mother Tantra*, one of the most important of the Bön texts, offers us examples, similes, and metaphors to ponder in order to better understand this illusory nature of both dream and waking life:

Reflection. The dream is a projection of the mind. It is not different from the mind, just as a ray of sunlight is not different from the light of the sun in the sky. Not knowing this, we engage the dream as if it were real, like a lion snarling at the face it sees reflected in water. In a dream everything we experience is the mind reflected back at us.

Lightning. In the night sky, lightning flashes. Suddenly the mountains are illuminated, each peak seemingly a separate object. But what we are experiencing is a single flash of light being reflected back to our eyes. Just so, the seemingly separate objects in a dream are actually reflections of the single light of the mind, the light of awareness.

Rainbow. Like a rainbow, the dream can be beautiful and alluring. But it has no substance; it is a display of light and depends on the perspective of the observer. If we chase it, we can never reach it; there is nothing there. The dream, like the rainbow, is a combination of conditions from which an illusion arises.

Moon. The dream is like a moon reflected in many different waters—in the pond, the well, the sea—and in many different windows in a town and in many different crystals. The moon is not multiplying. There is only one moon, just as the many objects of a dream are of one essence.

Magic. A magician can make a single stone appear first as an elephant, then as a snake, then as a tiger. But these objects are illusory. Like the objects in a dream, they are projections of the light of the mind.

Mirage. Due to secondary causes, we may see a mirage in a desert, a shimmering city, or a lake. But when we approach, we find nothing there. When we investigate the images of a dream, they, like the mirage, are found to be insubstantial illusions, the play of light.

Echo. If we make a loud sound where there are conditions for echoes, a loud sound returns to us; a quiet sound returns a quiet sound;

and a strange cry comes back to us as a strange cry. The sound we hear returning is the sound we made, just as the content of a dream appears to be independent of us but is only the projected content of the mind returning to us.

These examples stress the lack of inherent existence in appearances. In the sutric teachings, we call this "emptiness"; in tantra, "illusion"; and in Dzogchen, "the single sphere." The self and the object of experience are not two. We experience the world within and without in our minds. If we dissolve the conceptual mind, the underlying purity manifests spontaneously. When we directly know there is no inherent existence, neither in the self or the world, then whatever arises as experience has no power over us. When the lion understands the illusory nature of the reflection in the water, he does not react with fear.

Teaching Metaphors

The *Mother Tantra* says the ignorance of ordinary sleep is like a dark room. Awareness is the flame of a lamp. When the lamp is lit, even if the room has been without light for centuries, darkness is dispelled and the room is illuminated.

I wanted to add this note about how to best work with metaphors and symbolic images as sometimes students have a problem with them. Using language and images to evoke experience, as poetry does, can be more useful in the teachings than explanations confined to abstract concepts. Images help when they are perceived by more than just the rational mind. They are to be experienced: pondered in the imagination, felt, and integrated into understanding.

For instance, when we hear the word "fire," we may pay little attention. But dwelling on it, allowing the image to emerge from behind the word, we see fire, we know the heat. Because we have all watched flame and felt the heat of it on our skin, if we stay with the image for a bit, the word evokes an imaginal experience we can almost feel. A fire burns in our imagination. Similarly, if we say "lemon" and let the fruit emerge from the word, our mouths water. When metaphors and symbols are used in the teaching, it is best to allow them to affect us this way. Use your imagination to know the experience hidden in the words and relate it to the teaching.

There is darkness. A lamp is lit. We all know this experience of a light being turned on. The darkness is replaced by luminosity that is clear, insubstantial but directly known. A wind arises, and the flame is blown out. We know what it feels like when light is overcome by darkness.

We must go beyond the image, but it can point us in the right direction.

PART TWO

Kinds and Uses of Dreams

The goal of dream practice is to realize what is beyond dreams altogether. But there are also uses of dream that are beneficial in everyday life. These include both using information we bring back from dreams and directly benefiting from experiences we have in dreams. In the West, for example, the use of dream therapy is widespread, and there are many accounts of artists and scientists using the creativity of dreams to benefit their work. Tibetans also rely on dreams in various ways. This section describes some of these uses of dreams.

CHAPTER 6

Three Kinds of Dreams

Three types of dream form a progression in dream practice, although not an exact one: (1) ordinary samsaric dreams, (2) dreams of clarity, and (3) clear light dreams. The first two types are distinguished by their different causes. In both, the dreamer may be either lucid or nonlucid. In clear light dreams, there is awareness but no subject-object dichotomy. Clear light dreams occur in nondual awareness.

Samsaric Dreams

Most of us generally have samsaric dreams arising from karmic traces and usually initiated by an experience in the day or the recent past: an interaction, an emotion or a thought, an image or a memory. Meaning found in these dreams is meaning we project into them; it is imputed by the dreamer rather than being inherent to the dream. This is also the case with meaning in waking life. This does not make meaningful dreams unimportant any more than it makes the meaning in waking life unimportant. The process is similar to reading a book. A book is just words printed on paper, but because we bring our sense of meaning to it, we can take meaning from it. And the meaning of a book, like that of a dream, is subject to interpretation. Two people can read the same book and have entirely different experiences—one person may change their whole life based on the meaning they found in the pages, while their friend may find the book only mildly interesting or not even that. The book has not changed. The meaning is projected onto the words by the reader and then read back.

Ordinary dreaming (Arises from personal karmic traces)	Nonlucid or lucid
Dreams of clarity (Arise from transpersonal karmic traces)	Nonlucid or lucid
Clear light dreams (Nonduality; no subject-object duality)	Lucid

Dreams of Clarity

As progress is made in dream practice, greater awareness is brought into the dream. Dreams become clearer and more detailed, and more dreams are remembered. Beyond this increased awareness in ordinary dreams is a second kind of dream called the dream of clarity. Such dreams arise when mind and prana are balanced as the dreamer develops the capacity to remain in aware presence. Unlike the samsaric dream, in which the mind is swept here and there by karmic prana, in the dream of clarity the dreamer is stable. Though the dream is still dualistic, images and information arise based less on personal karmic traces and situations. Instead, transpersonal knowledge is available; it's as if something is given to or found by the dreamer, as opposed to the samsaric dream in which meaning is projected by the dreamer into the dream experience.

Dreams of clarity are valued in many spiritual traditions. They seem to arise from the clearest, most open dimension of the dreamer. Shamanic and religious traditions record dreams in which a diagnosis is revealed or a healing occurs, life-changing insights are recognized, or prophecies and teachings are received. In modern times, many scientists have found the answer to a problem in a dream, artists have discovered new directions, and writers have found new plots.

Dreams of clarity may occasionally arise for anyone, but they are not common until practice is developed and stable. For most of us, all dreams are samsaric based on our daily lives and emotions. Even though we may have a dream about the teachings, our teachers, our practice, buddhas, or *dakinis*, the dream is still likely to be a samsaric dream. If we are involved in practice and a tradition, then we will dream about these things. It is a positive sign because it means that we are engaged in the teachings, but the engagement itself is dualistic and therefore in the realm of samsara. There are better and worse aspects of samsara, and it is good to be fully engaged in practice and the teachings because that is the path to liberation. It is also good not to mistake samsaric dreams for dreams of clarity.

If we make the mistake of believing samsaric dreams are offering us reliable guidance, then changing our lives daily while trying to follow the dictates of dreams can become a full-time job. It is also a way to become stuck in personal drama, believing all our dreams are messages from a higher, more spiritual source. It is not like that. We should pay close attention to dreams and develop some understanding of which have import and which are only manifestations of emotions, desires, fears, hopes, and fantasies.

Clear Light Dreams

A third type of dream occurs when one is far along the path: the clear light dream. It arises from the primordial prana in the central channel. The clear light is generally spoken of in the teachings about sleep yoga and indicates a state free from dream, thought, and image, but there is also a clear light dream in which the dreamer remains in the nature of mind. This is not an easy accomplishment; the practitioner must be stable in awareness before the clear light dream arises. Gyalshen Milu Samleg, the author of important commentaries on the *Mother Tantra*, wrote that he practiced consistently for nine years before he began to have clear light dreams.

Developing the capacity for clear light dreams is similar to developing the capacity of abiding in clear presence during the day. In the beginning, even after you have experience of rigpa, when you speak, you lose the connection to the underlying silence. When you move, you lose the connection to stillness. When you make a plan or attend to thought, you lose the experience of the spaciousness of awareness. But when stability in rigpa is developed, thought simply arises and dissolves without obscuring rigpa. Then you can speak, move, and be creative while abiding in clear presence.

When learning to play the drum and bell together in ritual practice, we can only do one at a time in the beginning. If we play the bell, we lose the rhythm of the drum, and vice versa. After we are stable, we can play both at the same time. This is similar to integrating activity and clear awareness; it takes practice.

The clear light dream is not the same as the dream of clarity, which, while arising from deep and relatively pure aspects of the mind, still takes place in duality. The clear light dream, while emerging from the karmic traces of the past, does not result in dualistic experience. The practitioner does not reconstitute as an observing subject in the world of the dream but abides wholly integrated with rigpa.

Samsaric dream arises from the individual's karmic traces and emotions, and all content of the dream is formed by those traces and emotions. The dream of clarity includes more objective knowledge, which arises from transpersonal karmic traces and is available to the consciousness when it is not entangled in personal karmic traces. The consciousness is then not bound by space, time or personal history, and the dreamer can meet with beings, receive teaching, and find information helpful to others as well as to themself.

The clear light dream is not defined by the content of the dream. It is a clear light dream because there is no subjective dreamer or dream ego, there is no self in relationship with the dream content. Although a dream arises, it is an activity of the mind that does not disturb the practitioner's stability in clear light.

CHAPTER 7

Uses of Dreams

The greatest value of dreams is in the context of the spiritual journey. They may provide experiences that motivate the dreamer to enter the spiritual path and may later be a means of determining whether the practice is being done correctly, how much progress is being made, and what needs attention. Most importantly, they can be used as a spiritual practice in themselves

As I said in the preface to the first edition, it is often the case that before giving a high teaching, the teacher will wait for the student to have a dream indicating their readiness to receive the teaching. Other dreams may demonstrate that the student has accomplished a certain practice, and after hearing the dream, the teacher may determine it is time for the student to move on to another practice.

If we pay attention to dreams, we can gauge our own maturity in the practice. Sometimes in the waking state we think we are doing quite well, but when we sleep, we find that at least some part of us is still greatly confused or stuck in negativity. This should not be discouraging. It is a benefit when different aspects of the mind manifest in dream and point out what we need to bring into the practice.

When practice becomes strong, the results of the practice will manifest in dream and give us confidence in our efforts.

Experience in Dreams

Experience is very flexible in dreams, and we are free to do a great many things we cannot do when we are awake. This includes specific practices to facilitate our development. We can heal wounds in the psyche, emotional difficulties that we have not been able to overcome. We can remove energetic blocks that may be inhibiting the free circulation of energy in the body. And we can pierce obscurations in the mind by taking experience beyond conceptual boundaries and limitations.

Generally, these tasks are best accomplished after we develop lucidity in dreams. It is mentioned here only as a possibility. In the section on practice, there is more detail about how to practice in a dream once lucidity is attained.

Guidance and Guidelines

Most Tibetans—high spiritual masters and simple, ordinary people—consider dreams to be a potential source of both profound spiritual knowledge and guidance for everyday life. Dreams are consulted to diagnose illness, for indications that practices of purification or clarification are needed, or that relationships to deities and guardians need attention. Such uses of dreams may be viewed as superstitious, but on a profound level, dreams portray the state of the dreamer and the condition of their relationship to different energies. In the East, people recognize these energies and relate to them as guardians and protector spirits as well as physiological, mental, and spiritual conditions. In Western psychology, much of this is not accepted, but dreams are examined for emotional or situational problems, suppressed psychic material, incipient illnesses, and the activity of archetypes. Dreams are also appreciated as a source of pleasure and creativity.

Some Tibetans work with dreams throughout their lives as a primary form of communication with deeper aspects of themselves and with other worlds. My mother was a good example of this. She was a practitioner and a very loving and kind woman. Often she told the whole family her dreams in the morning when we were gathered to eat, and particularly when the dream had to do with her guardian and protector, Namthel Karpo.

Namthel is a guardian of the northern part of Tibet, Hor, where my mother grew up. Although his practice was known throughout Tibet, he was particularly important in the village in which she lived and in the surrounding area. My mother did his practice, but my father did not, and often he would tease her after she recounted her dreams.

I clearly remember my mother telling us one dream in which Namthel came to her. He was dressed, as always, in white robes and conch-shell earrings, and he had long hair. This time he looked furious. He came through the door and roughly threw a little bag on the floor. He said, "I always tell you to take care of yourself, but you don't do a good job of it!" He looked deeply into my mother's eyes and then disappeared.

In the morning my mother was uncertain about the dream's meaning. But in the afternoon, a lady who sometimes worked in our home tried to steal our money. She was carrying it tucked under her clothes, but when she walked in front of my mother, the money fell out right there. It was in a bag identical to the one my mother had been shown in the dream. My mother picked it up, and inside was all of our money. She considered this event an activity of protection on the part of her guardian and believed Namthel caused the bag to fall to the floor.

Namthel appeared in my mother's dreams throughout her life, always in the same form. Though the messages he gave her varied, they were generally dreams meant to help her in some way, to protect her and guide her.

Until I was ten years old, I was in a Christian school, after which my parents took me out and I entered Menri Monastery. One of the monks, Gen Sengtuk, would sometimes tell me his dreams. I remember some of them clearly as they were similar to my mother's. He often dreamt of Sidpé Gyalmo, one of the most important and ancient of the enlightened protectors of the Bön tradition though her practice is also known in the other Tibetan Buddhist schools. In the Potala Palace in Tibet, there is a room housing her shrine. Gen Sengtuk's dreams of her guided him in life and practice.

Sidpé Gyalmo did not appear in his dreams as the ferocious being that we see in the paintings in temples and meditation rooms. Instead, he saw her as a very old, gray-haired human woman, in a body no longer straight, using a walking stick. Gen Sengtuk always met her in a vast desert where she had a tent. No one else lived there. The monk would read her expressions, whether her face was happy or sad, or if there was anger in the way she moved. Reading her this way, he would somehow know what to do to heal obstacles in his practice or to change certain things in his life in a more positive direction. This is how she guided him through dreams. He kept a close connection to her this way, and she appeared to him in a similar manner throughout his life. His experiences with her are good examples of dreams of clarity.

I was a little boy then, but I remember one day when, listening to the monk recounting one of his dreams, it suddenly struck me that it was as if he had a friend in a different place. I thought it would be nice to have some friends to play with in dreams; during the day, I could not play much as the studies were very intensive and the teachers strict. That was the thought I had then. So you see, our understanding of dream and dream practice—and our motivation to do the practice—can deepen and mature as we grow.

Divination

Many meditation masters, because of the stability of their meditation practice, are able to use dreams of clarity for divination. To do so, the dreamer must be able to free themself from most of the personal karmic traces that normally shape the dream. Otherwise, information is not obtained from the dream but is projected onto the dream, as is normally the case with samsaric dreams. In the Bön tradition, this use of dreams is considered one of several methods of shamanic divination and it is quite common among Tibetans. It is not unusual for a student to ask their teacher for guidance regarding an undertaking or for direction in overcoming an obstacle. Often the teacher turns to dreams to find the answer for the student.

For example, when I was in Tibet, I met a realized Tibetan woman named Khachod Wangmo. She was very powerful and a treasure finder (*terton*) who had rediscovered many hidden teachings. I asked her for knowledge of my future, a general question about obstacles I would encounter and so on. I asked her to have a dream of clarity for me.

Commonly in this situation, the dreamer asks for a possession of the person requesting the dream. I gave Khachod Wangmo the undershirt I was wearing. The shirt represented me energetically, and by focusing on it, she was able to connect to me. She put it under her pillow that night and had a dream of clarity. In the morning, she gave me a long explanation of what was to come in my life, things I should avoid and things I should do. It was clear and helpful guidance.

Sometimes a student asks whether a dream telling us something about the future means the future is fixed. In the Tibetan tradition, we believe it is not. The causes of all things that can happen are already present, right now. How we reacted to life in the past and how we react now plant seeds that condition our future experience. But the secondary causes necessary for the manifestation of the karmic seeds are not fixed; they are circumstantial. That is why practice is effective and why illness can be cured; we can alter karmic conditioning enough that when we encounter the secondary cause, we can choose to respond wisely rather than react from prior conditioning. If we have a dream about tomorrow and tomorrow comes and everything happens just as it did in our dream, this does not mean the future is fixed and cannot be changed; it means we didn't change it.

I remember an example of this from when I was young. It was a day called Diwali in India, traditionally celebrated with firecrackers. My friends and I didn't have money to buy firecrackers, so we looked for ones that had been lit but hadn't exploded. We gathered them and then tried to relight them. I was very young, four or five years old. One of the firecrackers was a little wet, and I put it on a burning coal. I shut my eyes and blew on it, and of course it exploded.

For a moment I couldn't see anything except stars, and right then I remembered my dream of the night before. It was exactly the same, the whole experience. In the dream, the karmic traces led to the recklessness I felt as a young boy. The secondary condition was the celebration the next day. It would have been much more helpful if I had remembered the dream before rather than after the event! If I had, I might have chosen to be more careful, and the dream would have seemed false while actually stimulating me to change the way I acted. There are many cases like this, in which the causes of future situations are woven into a dream about a future that is likely to, but will not necessarily, unfold.

Sometimes in a dream the causes and results affecting other people can be known. When I was in Tibet, my teacher, Lopon Tenzin Namdak, had a dream and then told me it was very important that I do a particular practice connected with one of the guardians. I began to do the practice for many hours every day while I traveled, trying to influence whatever he had seen in his dream. A few days after his dream, I was a passenger in a truck traveling on a tiny road high in the mountains. The drivers in that part of Tibet are wild, nomadic people with little fear of death. Thirty of us were crowded into a big truck with a lot of heavy luggage when the tire hit a hole and the truck tipped over.

I got out and looked down. I was not particularly afraid. But then I saw that one stone held the truck up, preventing it from sliding down into a valley, a drop so deep that a rock tossed over the edge took what seemed to be a long while to reach bottom. Then my heart started to bang around in my chest! I felt the fear, noticing that one stone was all that stood between us and death, that kept my life from ending as a short story.

When I saw what the situation was, I thought, "That's it. That's why I had to do the practice of the guardian." That was what my teacher had seen in his dream and why he told me to do the practice. A dream may not be very specific but can still convey the feeling and images of the dream that something is coming that needs to be addressed. This is one benefit we can receive from working with our dreams.

Teachings in Dreams

There are numerous examples in the Tibetan traditions of practitioners receiving teachings in dreams. Often the dreams come in sequence, each night's dream starting where the previous night's dream ends, in this way transmitting entire, detailed teachings until a precise and appropriate point of completion is reached. Then the dream sequence stops. Volumes of teachings have been "discovered" this way, including many of the practices that Tibetans have been engaging in for centuries. This is what we call "mind treasure" (*gong-ter*).

Imagine entering a cave and finding a volume of teachings hidden inside. This is finding in a physical space. Mind treasures are found in consciousness rather than in the physical world. Masters have been known to find these treasures both in dreams of clarity and when awake. To receive this kind of teaching in a dream, the practitioner must have developed certain capacities, such as being able to stabilize in awareness without identifying with the conventional self. The practitioner whose clarity is unobscured by karmic traces and samsaric dreams has access to wisdom inherent to clear awareness.

Authentic teachings discovered in dreams do not come from the intellect. It is not like going to the library and doing research and then writing a book, using the intellect to collect and synthesize information as a scholar might. Although many important teachings come from the intellect, they are not considered mind treasures. The wisdom of the buddhas is self-originated, rising from the depths of consciousness, complete in itself. This does not mean that mind treasure teachings will not resemble existing teachings; they will. These teachings can be found in different cultures and different historical periods and can be similar even though they do not inform each other. Historians work to trace a teaching back in time to point out how it was influenced by a similar teaching, where the historical connection took place, and so on, and often they find these links. But the underlying truth is that these teachings arise spontaneously from humans when they reach a certain point in their development, and that is true in various cultures and times. The teachings are inherent in the foundational wisdom of primordial awareness that any culture can eventually access. They are not only Buddhist or Bön teachings; they are the wisdom teachings of humanity.

If we have the karma to help other beings, the teachings from a dream may be of benefit to others. But it may also be the case, if we have karma with a lineage for example, that the teachings discovered in a dream will be particularly for our own practice, perhaps as a specific remedy to overcome an obstacle.

CHAPTER 8

The Discovery of Chöd Practice

Many masters of the past used dream as an important wisdom door through which they discovered teachings, made connections to masters who were otherwise distant in time and space, and developed the capacity to help others. All of these are illustrated in the story of Tongjung Thuchen, a great master of Bön. He is believed to have lived in the eighth century. In a series of dreams, he discovered the Bön practice of *chöd*, a visionary practice for cultivating generosity and cutting through attachment.

By the time Tongjung Thuchen was six years old, he was already knowledgeable about the teachings. At twelve he was making long retreats and having remarkable dream experiences in which he discovered teachings and met and received teachings from other masters. Once, when he was in a retreat and intensively doing the practice of Walsai, one of the important tantric deities of Bön, he was summoned by his master. He left the retreat and journeyed to the house of one of his master's sponsors where his master was staying.

The night he arrived, he dreamt that a beautiful woman led him through unknown landscapes until they came to a large cemetery. Many corpses lay on the ground. In the center stood a large white tent covered with ornate decorations and surrounded by beautiful flowers. In the center of the tent, a brown woman sat on a large throne. She wore a white dress, and her hair was ornamented with turquoise and gold. Many dakinis were gathered around her, speaking the languages of many different countries and leading Tongjung Thuchen to understand that they were from distant lands.

Leaving her throne, the brown dakini brought Tongjung Thuchen a skull full of blood and flesh and fed him from it. As she did, she told him to accept the offerings as pure offerings in preparation for an important initiation she and the other dakinis were going to give him.

Then she said, "May you achieve enlightenment in the space of the Great Mother. I am Sidpé Gyalmo, the holder of the Bön teaching, the Brown Queen of Existence. This initiation-teaching is the quintessential root *Mother Tantra*. I initiate you so that you can initiate and teach this to others." Tongjung Thuchen was led to a high throne. After Sidpé Gyalmo gave him a ceremonial hat, an initiation robe, and ritual implements, she surprised him by requesting that he give initiation to the gathered dakinis.

Tongjung Thuchen said, "Oh no, I can't give initiation. I don't know how to do this. I am very embarrassed."

Sidpé Gyalmo reassured him. "Don't worry. You are a great master. You have all the initiations from the thirty masters of Tibet and Zhang Zhung. You can give us initiation."

"But I don't know how to sing the prayers during the initiation," Tongjung Thuchen protested.

Sidpé Gyalmo said, "I'll help you and all the protectors will give you power. There is nothing to be afraid of. Please perform the initiation."

At that point, all of the meat and blood in the tent transformed into butter, sugar, various foodstuffs, medicine, and flowers. The dakinis tossed flowers on him. Suddenly he realized that he did know how to give the initiation for the *Mother Tantra*, and he did so.

Afterward the dakinis thanked him. Sidpé Gyalmo said, "In five years the dakinis from the eight major cemeteries will meet, as will many masters. If you come, we will give you more teachings from the *Mother Tantra*."

The dakinis and Tongjung Thuchen said their farewells, and Sidpé Gyalmo told him he was to leave. A red dakini wrote a YAM syllable on a scarf, representing the wind element, waved it in the air, and asked him to touch the scarf with his right foot. The moment he did, he was back in his body, aware that he was sleeping.

He slept for a such a long time that his hosts were afraid he was dead. When he finally woke, his master asked him why he had slept so long. He recounted the dream to his master, who told him that it was quite wonderful but also cautioned him to keep it secret lest it become an obstacle. The master told Tongjung Thuchen that someday he would be a teacher and then gave him a blessing to empower his future teachings.

The following year, Tongjung Thuchen was in retreat when one evening he was visited by three dakinis. They had green scarves, which they touched to his feet. As they did so, he lost consciousness briefly, then woke in a dream.

He saw three caves facing east. A beautiful lake was in front of the caves. He walked into the central cave. Inside, it was wonderfully decorated with flowers. He met three masters, each dressed differently in esoteric initiation clothes. They were surrounded by dakinis, who played musical instruments, danced, made offerings, prayed, and performed other sacred activities.

The three masters gave him initiations to wake him to the natural state, to cause him to remember his past lives, and to enable him to teach the chöd practice successfully. The central master stood and said, "You have all the sacred teachings. You have received the initiations, and we have blessed you to empower your ability to teach."

The master who sat to the right rose and said, "We initiate you into all the general teachings, the logical philosophies used to cut the ego, the use of the conceptual mind to liberate delusions, and the chöd practices. We bless you so you can teach these practices and give them continuity."

The master on the left stood and said, "I'm going to give you the sacred tantric teaching that is at the heart of all the masters of Tibet and Zhang Zhung. We initiate you and bless you through these teachings so you can help others."

All three masters were important Bön masters who had lived around the end of the seventh century, more than five hundred years before Tongjung Thuchen was born.

Sometime later, after Tongjung Thuchen's master passed away, Tongjung Thuchen returned to his master's little village and did rituals and practices for the people there. On numerous occasions, during both short meditations and retreats, he was visited by various masters in visions. He experienced being able to see inside his own body, where the channels and energies appeared as clear crystal. Many times when he walked, his feet did not touch the ground, and he could walk very, very fast using the power of his prana.

Four more years passed. The brown dakini from his dream, the manifestation of Sidpé Gyalmo, had told him they would meet again after five years, and the time had arrived. One day he took a nap in a cave and during sleep prayed to all the masters. When he awoke, he looked into a perfectly clear sky. A small breeze arose, and two dakinis came to him, riding the wind, and told him he was to accompany them.

He went with them to a gathering of dakinis, the same dakinis from many lands whom he had met in the dream five years earlier. He received transmissions and explanations of the chöd practices and the *Mother Tantra*. The dakinis predicted a future time during which bodhisattvas and twelve blessed masters would appear and Tongjung Thuchen would teach. Each dakini made a promise to aid him in teaching. One said that she would act as a guardian of the teachings, another said she would bless the teachings, the next that she would protect the teachings from erroneous words and interpretations, and so on. Sidpé Gyalmo pledged to act as a protector of the teachings. In turn, each of the assembled dakinis told him what responsibilities she would undertake to aid the dissemination of the teachings. They told him the teachings would spread in the ten directions like the rays of the sun, to all the areas of the world. That prophecy was an important one and encourages those who today learn these practices, because we know they are spreading across the earth.

Tongjung Thuchen's dreams are good examples of dreams of clarity. He received accurate information in one dream regarding an important dream he would have in the future. He received teachings and initiations and was aided by dakinis and other masters. In the early part of his life, though he was accomplished, he did not know his full potential until it was revealed to him in a dream. Through the blessings he received in dreams, he woke to different dimensions of consciousness and was reconnected to the part of himself that had learned and developed in past lives. He continued growing through his dreams, receiving teachings and meeting with masters and dakinis throughout his life.

So it can be for all of us. We will find, as practitioners, a continuity developing in the part of our lives we spend in dreams. This is valuable in our spiritual journey. Dream becomes part of a process that reconnects us to our deeper selves and matures our spiritual development.

CHAPTER 9

Two Levels of Practice

One night, many years ago, I dreamed a snake was in my mouth. I pulled it out and found it was dead. It was quite unpleasant. An ambulance arrived at my house. The paramedics told me the snake was poisonous and that I was dying. I said, "Okay."

They took me to the hospital. I was afraid and told them I needed to see a statue of Tapihritsa, the Dzogchen master, before I died. The paramedics did not know who he was, but they agreed with my request and told me I would have to wait to die, which relieved me. But then they surprised me by bringing the statue right away. My excuse for delaying death had not worked for very long. So I told them there was no death; this was now my crutch. The minute I said that, I awoke with a rapidly beating heart.

It was New Year's Eve, and the next day I was to fly to Rome from Houston. Feeling uncomfortable after the dream, I thought perhaps I should take it seriously and cancel my travel plans. I wanted my teacher's advice. So I went back to sleep and, in a lucid dream, traveled to Lopon in Nepal and told him of the disturbing dream.

At that time, Houston was having a lot of trouble with flooding. My teacher interpreted the dream to mean that I was representing the *garuda*, the mystical bird who has power over the *nagas*, the snakelike water spirits. Lopon said the dream meant that the garuda was conquering the water spirits who were causing the flooding. This interpretation made me feel much better. The next day I went to Rome as planned. This is an example of using lucid dream for something practical, for making decisions.

This may all sound strange and unbelievable. The real point is to develop the flexibility of the mind and to pierce the boundaries constricting it. With greater flexibility, we can better accept what arises without being influenced by expectations and desires. Even while we are still limited by grasping and aversion, this kind of spiritual practice will benefit our daily lives.

If I am truly living in the realization that there is no death and no one to die, then I will not seek interpretation of a dream as I did in this case, when the dream left me feeling anxious. Our desire for interpretation of a dream is based on hope and fear; we want to know what to avoid and what to promote, we want to obtain understanding in order to change something. When you realize your true nature, you do not need to seek meaning. You are then beyond hope and fear and the meaning of a dream becomes unimportant; you simply experience fully whatever manifests in the present moment. No dream, then, can cause anxiety.

Dream yoga spans the whole of our lives and applies to all dimensions of experience. This can lead to a sense of conflict between the highest philosophical view and some of the instructions. On the one hand, the view is boundless; the teachings of nonduality and nonconventional reality declare there is nothing to accomplish, that seeking is losing, that effort carries one away from one's true nature. On the other hand, there are practices and teachings that only make sense in terms of hope and fear. Instruction is given on interpreting dreams, pacifying local guardians, and accomplishing long-life practices, and the student is urged to practice with diligence and guard the focus of the mind. It seems we are being told both that there is nothing to accomplish and that we need to work very hard.

Sometimes this contradiction leads a practitioner into confusion regarding practice. The question arises: "If ultimate reality is empty of distinctions, and if liberation is to be found in the realization of this empty nature, then why should I do practices aimed at relative results?" The answer is simple. Because we live in a dualistic, relative world, we do practices effective in this world. In samsaric existence, dichotomies and polarities have meaning; there is right and wrong and better and worse ways to act and think based on the values of different religions, spiritual schools, philosophical systems, science, and culture. Respect the circumstances in which you are bound. When living in samsara, conventional practices apply, and dream interpretation can be very helpful.

In our conventional lives, we make choices and can change things; that is why we study the teachings, why we practice. As we understand more and become more skilled in our lives, we become more flexible. We begin to really understand the things we are taught: what lucidity is, what is illusory about our experiences, how suffering comes about, what our true nature is. Once we start to see how what we do is a cause of suffering, we can choose to do something different. We grow weary of constricted identities and the repetitive inclinations that lead to so much unnecessary suffering. We let go of negative emotional states, train ourselves to overcome distraction, and abide in pure presence.

It is the same with dreaming. There is a progression in the practice. As the practice is developed, we discover there is another way to dream. Then we move toward the unconventional dream practices in which the story and its interpretations are not important. We work more on the causes of dreams than the dreams themselves.

There is no reason not to use dream yoga to attain worldly goals. Some of the practices address relative concerns and lead to the use of dreaming for purposes such as health, divination, guidance, cleansing unhealthy karmic and psychological tendencies, healing, and so on. The path is practical and suited for all. But while the use of dream yoga to benefit us in the relative world is good, it is a provisional use of the practice.

I needed the interpretation of my snake dream because I was afraid of death. It is important for me to know my need was based on fear and that when I abide in nondual presence, there is no fear and I need no interpretation. We use what is useful for the situation in which we find ourselves. When we live only in the nature of mind, the state in which reality truly is void of distinctions, we do not need to do relative practices. There is no need for the interpretation of dream because there is no need to redirect ourselves, there is no egoic self to redirect. We do not need to consult a dream about the future because there is no hope or fear related to the future. We do not need to look to the dream for meaning. We are completely present in whatever arises, without aversion or attraction, because we are living in the truth.

PART THREE

The Practice of Dream Yoga

CHAPTER 10

Vision, Action, Dream, Death

If one is not aware in vision,
One will not be aware in behavior.
If one is not aware in behavior,
One will not be aware in dream.
If one is not aware in dream,
One will not be aware in the bardo of death.

The Mother Tantra (Ma Gyud)

"Vision" in this context does not mean only visual phenomena. Vision is every perception, sensation, thought, and emotion appearing in consciousness: the totality of experience.

Being unaware in vision means being deluded, mistaking the projections and fantasies of the moving mind for reality and living in that illusion.

Pushed this way and that by desire and aversion, striving for pleasure and trying to avoid pain, our conditioning determines our reactions to what we encounter outside and in our minds. This is being unaware in action, in behavior.

For example, someone says something negative; they attack you, challenge you, hurt you, or reject you. You are immediately caught up in your story and react from conditioning, growing angry or defensive or hurt. You lose connection to clear awareness; you don't have the sense of spaciousness inside. You lose yourself in the waking dream. This is first being unaware in vision; then reacting without full awareness is being unaware in behavior.

When, in meditation or in daily life, you are stable in clear aware-ness, you are whole. You are complete. When you experience some-thing from outside, you are not shaken. You just let experience arise. You don't feel threatened or hurt because you recognize the dreamlike nature of the interaction. When someone says something negative, you hear it, you listen, you let it go. This is being aware in vision.

When you abide in the peace of clear awareness, you can feel compassion for the attacker, you see the person is lost in their own dream. You can respond with care; you don't need to win the dis-agreement. This is being aware in action, being aware in behavior.

Dreams in sleep arise from the same conditioning that governs our waking experience. If we are too distracted to penetrate the fantasies and delusions of the moving mind during the day, we will likely be bound by the same limitations in dream. Dream phenom-ena will evoke in us the same emotions and reactions in which we are lost when awake, even if we are lucid in the dream, making it difficult to develop the lucidity and engage in further practices. This is not being aware in dream.

As we practice dream yoga, we continually bring awareness to the immediate moment of experience while awake. As we develop consistency, this lucidity will be found in dream. While awake and paying attention to the moment, we practice skillfully responding to what arises. Eventually we will be able to do the same in dream. There will be more lucidity, more skillful responses to what arises, more ability to transform the situations and our identities. This is being aware in dream.

We enter the bardo, the intermediate state after death, as we enter dream after falling asleep. If our experience of dream lacks clarity and is of confused emotional states and habitual reactivity, we will have trained ourselves to experience the processes of death in the same way. We react dualistically and unconsciously to the visions that arise in the intermediate state: the images, the emotions, the feelings. Our future rebirth will be determined by the karmic tenden-cies we have cultivated in life. This is lacking awareness in the bardo.

If you are aware in waking life and dream life, able to abide in clear awareness, you will not get lost in the story. You will have the capacity to reach liberation in death. This is being aware in the bardo.

So this is the sequence: awareness in the first moment of experience and in response to experience in waking life, in dream, and in death. We cannot start at the end. Three of these we can practice every day and night; death we can only practice once in this life.

Determine for yourself how mature your practice is. As you encounter the phenomena of your life, examine your reactions, your feelings and thoughts. Do your mind and heart remain open when you encounter something or someone you find unpleasant? Are you thrown into negative emotions by your attractions and aversions? Or can you remain in clear, steady presence in diverse situations? Dream yoga practice cultivates the stability in awareness needed to free yourself of conditioning and reactivity. Develop stability in lucidity during the day, and you will increasingly develop stability in awareness at night. Your dreams will change in extraordinary ways.

CHAPTER 11

Calm Abiding: Zhiné

All yogic and spiritual disciplines include some form of mind training to strengthen concentration and quiet the mind enough to remain undistracted in practice. In the Tibetan tradition, this practice is called calm abiding (zhiné). We recognize three stages in the development of stability: forceful zhiné, natural zhiné, and ultimate zhiné. Zhiné begins with mental fixation on an object. When concentration is strong enough, the practice moves to fixation without an object.

Begin the practice by sitting in the five-pointed meditation posture: legs crossed, hands folded in the lap in meditation position with palms up, one on top of the other. The spine is straight but not rigid, the head tilted down slightly to straighten the back of the neck, the eyes open. If the posture is too uncomfortable or impossible, sit in any posture that allows the spine to be straight, with the head slightly bent and the eyes open.

The eyes should be relaxed, not too wide open and not too closed. Place the object of concentration so as to allow the eyes to look straight ahead, neither up nor down. During the practice, try not to move, not even to swallow or blink, while keeping the mind one-pointedly on the object. Even if tears stream down your face, try not to move. Let the breathing be natural.

We generally use the Tibetan letter *A*, seen in the following images, as the object of concentration. This has many symbolic meanings, but here it is used simply as a support for the development of focus. Other objects may be used: the letter *A* of the

English alphabet, an image, the sound of a mantra, the breath—almost anything. However, it is good to use something connected to the sacred as it serves to inspire. If possible, use the same object each time you practice rather than switching between objects; the continuity supports the practice. It is also somewhat preferable to focus on a physical object outside the body because the purpose is to develop stability during the perception of external objects and, eventually, of the objects in dreams.

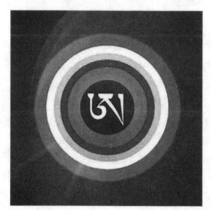

Tibetan *A*

If you choose to use the Tibetan *A*, download the image from the internet or draw it on a piece of paper about an inch square. Traditionally the letter is white, enclosed in five concentric colored circles: the center circle, the background for the *A*, is indigo; around it is a blue circle, then green, red, yellow, and white, but you can make it as simple as black on white paper. Tape the paper to a stick just long enough to support the paper at eye level when you sit for practice, and make a base that holds it upright. Or tape the image to the wall at eye level, about a foot and a half or two feet in front of your eyes, or where it is most comfortable for your gaze.

As concentration strengthens and periods of practice are extended, unusual sensations arise in the body and strange visual phenomena appear. You may find your mind doing strange things too. That's okay. These experiences are a natural part of the development of concentration; they arise as the mind settles. Be neither disturbed by nor excited about them.

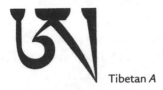

Tibetan *A*

Forceful Zhiné

The first stage of practice is called "forceful" because it requires effort. Normally, the mind is easily and quickly distracted. It may seem impossible to remain focused on the object for even a minute. In the beginning, rather than a long session, it is helpful to practice in numerous short sessions alternating with breaks. Do not let the mind wander during the break. Instead, recite a mantra; work with visualization; or engage in another practice you may know, such as the development of compassion. After the break, return to the fixation practice. If you are ready to practice but do not have the particular object you have been using, visualize a ball of light on your forehead and center yourself there. The practice should be done once or twice a day, or more frequently if you have time. Developing concentration is like strengthening the muscles of the body; exercising regularly and frequently works best. To become stronger, keep pushing against your limits.

Keep the mind on the object. Don't follow thoughts of the past or the future. Don't allow the attention to be carried away by fantasy, sound, physical sensation, or any other distraction. Just remain in the sensuality of the present moment. With strength and clarity, focus the mind on the object. Try not to lose awareness of the object for even a moment. Breathe gently, and then more gently, until the sense of breathing is lost. Slowly allow yourself to enter deeply into quiet and calm. Make certain the body is kept relaxed; don't tense up in concentration. Equally, don't allow yourself to fall into a stupor, a dullness, or a trance.

Don't think about the object, just let it be in awareness. This is an important distinction to make. Thinking about the object is not the kind of concentration we are developing. The point is just to keep the mind placed on the object, on the sense perception of the object, to undistractedly remain aware of the presence of the object. When the mind does get distracted—and it will again and again and again—gently bring it back to the object and rest there.

Natural Zhiné

As stability is developed, the second stage of practice is entered: natural zhiné. In the first stage, concentration is developed by continually directing the attention to the object and pacifying the unruly mind. In the second stage, the mind is absorbed in contemplation of the object; there is no longer the need for effort to hold it still. A relaxed and pleasant tranquility is established in which the mind is quiet. Thoughts arise without distracting the mind from the object. The elements of the body become harmonized, and the prana moves evenly and gently throughout the body. This is an appropriate time to move to fixation without an object.

Abandoning the physical object, simply fix the focus in space. It's helpful to gaze into expansive space, like the sky, but the practice can be done even in a small room by fixing on the space between your body and the wall. Remain steady and calm. Relaxation is key. Let go of any tension in your body. Rather than focusing on an imagined point in space, allow the mind, while remaining in strong presence, to be diffuse and awareness to be wide. Be aware of your entire visual field at once. We call this "dissolving the mind in space" or "merging the mind with space." It will lead to stable tranquility and the third stage of zhiné practice.

Ultimate Zhiné

Whereas in the second stage there is still some heaviness involved in the absorption in the object, the third stage is characterized by a mind that is tranquil but light, relaxed, and pliable. Thoughts arise and dissolve spontaneously and without effort.

In the Dzogchen tradition, this is when the master introduces the student to the natural state of mind. This is known as the "pointing out" instruction. Because the student has developed zhiné, the master is able to point to the nature of mind, which the student has experienced but not recognized. The pointing out helps the student to discriminate the moving mind, nearly always tangled with thoughts and concepts, from the nature of mind, which is pure, nondual awareness. This is the ultimate stage of zhiné practice, abiding in nondual presence, rigpa.

Obstacles

In developing zhiné practice, three obstacles must be overcome: agitation, drowsiness, and laxity.

Agitation

Agitation causes the mind to jump restlessly from one thought to another and makes concentration difficult. To prevent this, calm yourself before the practice session by avoiding too much physical or mental activity. Slow stretches may help to relax the body and quiet the mind. Once you are sitting, take a few deep, slow breaths. Make it a rule to focus the mind immediately when you start the practice to avoid developing the habit of mentally wandering while sitting in meditation posture.

Drowsiness

Drowsiness or sleepiness moves into the mind like a fog, a heaviness and torpor that blunts awareness. When it does, try to strengthen the mind's focus on the object in order to penetrate the drowsiness. You may find the drowsiness is actually a kind of movement of the mind that you can stop with strong concentration. If this doesn't work, take a break, stretch, and perhaps practice while standing.

Laxity

When encountering laxity, your mind may be calm but in a passive, weak mental state in which the concentration has no strength. It is important to recognize this state for what it is. It can be a pleasant and relaxed experience and, if mistaken for correct meditation, may lead to years spent mistakenly cultivating it, with no discernable change in the quality of consciousness. If your focus loses strength and your practice becomes lax, straighten your posture and wake up your mind. Reinforce the attention and guard the stability of presence. Regard the practice as something precious, which it is, and as something that will lead to the attainment of the highest realization, which it will. Strengthen intention and the wakefulness of the mind is automatically strengthened as well.

Daily Practice

Zhiné is best practiced every day until the mind is quiet and stable. Not only is it a preliminary practice, but it is helpful at any point in the practitioner's life. Even very advanced practitioners practice zhiné. The stability of mind developed through zhiné is the foundation of dream yoga and all other meditation practices. Once we have achieved a strong and reliable steadiness in calm presence, we can develop this in all aspects of life. When stable, this presence can always be found, and we will not be carried away by thoughts and emotions. Then, even though karmic traces continue to produce dream images after we fall asleep, we remain in awareness. This opens the door to the further practices of both dream and sleep yogas.

It's not necessary to attain ultimate zhiné in order to practice dream yoga, though if you did, the practice would be very easy. But you need enough stability of focus to remain lucid in a dream without being carried away by the story, just as you need some stability in waking life to keep from losing awareness and acting from habitual reactivity. Continuing to practice zhiné daily, even for only a few minutes here and there, is helpful as you start and continue the foundational and main practices.

CHAPTER 12

The Four Foundational Practices

Four foundational practices are the roots of dream yoga. Although traditionally called the Four Preparations, they are not of lesser importance, to be followed by the "real" practice. They are the essential practices, the foundation on which success in dream yoga depends.

The daily life of the mind determines the quality of our lives and the quality of our dreams. Change the way you experience your waking life and you change the experience of dream; the "you" that lives the dreams of waking life is the same "you" that lives the dreams of sleep. If you spend the day distracted, reacting to events and people from unconscious conditioning, then you are likely to do the same in dreams. If you are present and lucid when awake, you will eventually find that lucidity in dreams. It works in the other direction too; change the way you are in dreams and you change your waking life.

One: Changing the Karmic Traces

The practice is to repeatedly recognize the dreamlike nature of all experience, throughout the day, until the recognition manifests in dreams.

It begins upon waking. Think to yourself, "I am awake in a dream." Become fully present. Pay attention to the light in the room, sounds, sensations. When you enter the kitchen, recognize it as a dream kitchen. Pour dream milk into dream coffee. "It's a dream," you think. Drive a dream car to your dream job. Remind yourself of this frequently throughout the day.

The emphasis should be on you, the dreamer, more than on the objects of your experience. Keep reminding yourself you are dreaming up your experience: the irritation you feel, the happiness, the fatigue, the anxiety, the plans, the ruminations—all are part of the dream. The tree you appreciate, the people you meet, the places you visit—all part of the dream. You are creating a new habit of mind, new karma. It becomes part of your day to frequently, even if only for a moment, become intensely present and aware, to become lucid, dropping the stories being told in your mind and instead resting in vivid awareness.

When we think of experience as "only a dream," it loses power over us—power it only had because we gave it power. As we view life differently, we change our reaction to it. We can cut through our reactive conditioning. Our dreaming changes. But it's not just change in the dreams of the night. We begin to encounter all experience with greater calm and increased clarity. As the practice deepens, life becomes increasingly vivid, and appreciation and joy arise. Situations that were disturbing before are now seen as opportunities to practice.

When we say waking life, too, is a dream, it doesn't mean we can suddenly fly or transform into a lion. Instead, it's the realization that the entirety of experience takes place in the mind and that how we make meaning of an experience and react to it is due to our conditioning. This is one articulation of the realization that all phenomena are empty, that the apparent self-nature of beings and objects is illusory. There is not an actual "thing" anywhere in waking life—just as in a dream—but only transient appearances arising, changing, and dissolving. We are necessarily present when this realization comes, as it is then true that there is no place else to be. There is no stronger method of bringing consistent lucidity to dream than by abiding continuously in lucid presence during the day.

An important part of this practice is to experience yourself as a dream. Imagine yourself as a dream figure. Imagine your personality and various identities as constructions of mind. Maintain vivid presence, the same lucidity you are trying to cultivate in dreams, while sensing yourself as insubstantial and transient, made of light. This creates a very different relationship with yourself—one that is comfortable, flexible, and expansive.

It's not enough to simply repeat again and again that you are in a dream. Feel it. Is it true? Look, touch, smell, taste, listen. Is it a dream? Open your senses, as if this is your first moment of being in this world. When practiced correctly, each time you think you are in a dream, presence becomes stronger and experience brighter and more vivid. If there is not an immediate qualitative change in experience, check to make sure your practice isn't only the mechanical repetition of a phrase. There is no magic in just thinking a formula. When practicing the recognition, "wake" yourself—by increasing clarity and presence—again and again until just remembering the thought "This is a dream" opens the moment, quieting the moving mind if only for seconds.

There is an important warning regarding this practice. You must respect the logic, limitations, and responsibilities of conventional life. When you tell yourself waking life is a dream, this is true; but if you leap from a building, you will fall, not fly. If you quit work, bills will go unpaid. Plunge your hand in fire and it will be burned. It's of the utmost importance to remain grounded in the realities of the ordinary world, and it is a necessary part of the practice. As long as there is a "me" and an "other," there is a world in which we live and to which we are responsible. We are surrounded by suffering beings who benefit from our compassionate responses and who are harmed if we react without care or disregard their suffering as "only dream." Our decisions and actions have consequences. It's important to develop both the wisdom of seeing the empty, dreamlike nature of things and the compassion to respond to all that arises with generosity, kindness, and goodwill.

This is the first preparation: to recognize the dreamlike quality of life by developing the practice of lucid awareness. It is to be applied in the moment of perception, before a reaction arises. It is a potent practice in itself. Remain in this awareness and you will experience lucidity both while awake and during dreams. Lucidity in waking life and lucidity in dream are the same.

Two: Removing Grasping and Aversion

The second foundational practice works to decrease grasping and aversion.

The first foundational practice is applied in the immediate moment of encountering phenomena and before a reaction occurs. The second practice is engaged after a reaction has arisen. They are essentially the same practice, distinguished only by the situation in which they are applied and the object of attention. The first practice directs lucid awareness to the recognition of all phenomena of experience as dream. The second foundation specifically directs the same lucid awareness to emotionally shaded reactions that occur in response to the elements of experience.

Ideally the practice should be applied as soon as any grasping or aversion arises in response to an object or a situation. The grasping mind may manifest its reaction as desire, anger, jealousy, pride, envy, grief, despair, joy, anxiety, depression, fear, boredom, or any other emotion, whether intense or very subtle. This is in contrast to most reactions to phenomena, which are neutral.

When a reaction arises, become aware. Remind yourself that you, the person or object, and your reaction to the situation are all dream. Think to yourself, "This anger is a dream. This desire is a dream. This indignation/grief/exuberance is a dream." The truth in this statement becomes clear when you pay attention to the inner processes that produce emotional states: you literally dream them up through a complex interaction of thoughts, images, bodily states, and sensations. Emotional reactivity does not originate "out there" in objects. It arises, is experienced, and dissolves in your mind.

A limitless number of stimuli appear in life to which you may react: attraction may arise at the sight of a beautiful man or woman, anger at a driver cutting in front of you, disgust or sorrow at a ruined environment, anxiety and worry about a situation or person, and on and on. Every situation and reaction should be recognized as a dream. Do not just say, "It's a dream." Recognize and feel the dreamlike quality of your inner life. When this assertion is felt, not just thought, the relationship to the situation changes. The emotional grip on the object relaxes. The situation becomes clearer and more spacious. Grasping and aversion are directly recognized as the uncomfortable constrictions they are.

This is a powerful antidote to the state of near obsession generated from negative emotional states. Direct and certain experience of using this practice to untie the knots of negative emotion is the beginning of the deeper practice of lucidity and flexibility leading to freedom. With consistent practice, even strong experience of anger, depression, anxiety, and other states of unhappiness can be released. When they are, they dissolve. Instead of blindly reacting in a situation, you can respond with kindness, respect, and compassion. Each time you succeed, you plant another karmic seed, developing the habit of mind to respond positively to life. It will start to show up in dreams too.

The teachings refer to this particular practice as a method to give up attachments. There are healthy and unhealthy ways to go about this. It does one little good to suppress desires; they are then transformed into internal turmoil or external condemnations and intolerance. It also works against spiritual development to attempt to flee from pain through distraction or by tightening the body to choke off experience. It can be healthy to give up worldly life and become a monk or a nun, or it can be an unhealthy attempt to escape difficult experiences through suppression and avoidance.

Dream yoga cuts attachment by altering the view, we come to see objects and situations as empty, radiant and transient; like a dream. This diminishes grasping and aversion based on preference and supports equanimity.

Three: Strengthening Intention

The third foundation involves reviewing the day before going to sleep and strengthening the intention to practice during the night.

During the day, you've been practicing with vision and action, with experience and reactions to experience. Now, as you prepare for sleep, allow the memories of the day to arise. Was it a wonderful day? Neutral? Terrible?

Whatever comes to mind, recognize it as a dream. The memories most likely to arise are those of experiences that were strong enough to affect the coming dreams. During the day, which experience did you see as dream? Which captured you? The review can be short, seeing the whole of the day as a dream and remembering experiences briefly. Review the day as if you are remembering dreams; memory is very similar to dream.

This is a practice. Try to comprehend how you were caught up in the dreamlike nature of your life and the stories you tell about life. Feel the difference of relating to experience as a dream.

When experience becomes a memory, the memory often includes an emotional flavor. When we remember we may, to some extent, reexperience what we remember. Memories can make us happy, proud, grateful, loving, or nostalgic. Others we experience as painful, annoying, shameful, or frightening. In either case, memories affect us as they arise in consciousness.

By revisiting difficult memories while resting the mind in clear awareness, the memories lose their power to condition us. If we missed the opportunity to recognize the dreamlike nature of experiences during the day, we have another opportunity to do so in the evening review. The key is to remain relaxed in body and mind, and fully present. Recognize the memory as a dream. Simply witness the memory without engaging the story, then let it go.

After the review, develop the strongest intention possible to know directly and vividly, while dreaming, that you are dreaming. The intention is like an arrow directed at lucidity in dream, an arrow your mind follows. The Tibetan phrase we use for generating intention translates as "sending a wish." We should have that sense here, that we are making prayers and intentions and sending them to our teachers and to the buddhas and deities, promising to try to remain in awareness and asking for help. There are other practices that can be done before falling asleep, but this one is available to all.

Four: Cultivating Memory and Joyful Effort

The fourth foundational practice begins with waking in the morning. It further cultivates strong intention and strengthens the capacity to remember the events of the night.

Begin by reviewing the night. The Tibetan term for this is literally "remembering." Did you dream? Were you aware of being in a dream? If you dreamed but did not attain lucidity, reflect, "I dreamed but did not recognize the dream as a dream. But it was a dream." Resolve that next time you enter a dream, you will become aware of its nature while still in the dream.

If you find it difficult to remember dreams, it can be helpful, throughout the day and particularly before sleep, to generate a strong intention to remember dreams. One of the most helpful practices to increase dream recall is to record your dreams as soon as you wake. To make this easier, keep a journal, pen, and small light by your bed. Or use a recorder; most smartphones come with a recording app or you can download one. Keep this ready by your bedside. The very act of preparing the notebook or recorder at night serves to support the intention to recall the dream upon waking. It is not difficult for anyone to remember dreams once the intention to do so is generated and sustained, even over just a few days or weeks. The more dreams you record, the clearer your memory of dreams will become.

If you did have a lucid dream, feel joy. Develop happiness relative to the practice, and resolve to continue to develop lucidity the following night. If you weren't lucid, don't be discouraged. Instead, strengthen your determination, and know that the result will come if you continue the practice. Keep building intention, using both successes and failures as occasions to develop stronger intent to accomplish the practice.

Finally, during the morning period, generate a strong intention to remain consistent in practice throughout the day. Pray with your full heart for success. Prayer is like a magical power we all have and forget to use.

This practice merges into the first foundational practice, recognizing all experience as a dream. The practice becomes uninterrupted around the wheel of day and night.

Consistency

The importance of the day practices to the later stages of dream yoga cannot be overstated. They are much more powerful than they may appear to be. They are practices anyone can do. They are more psychologically oriented than many practices and present no difficulty for the practitioner. Simply doing a practice before going to bed may be ineffective, but with consistent practice of the foundational practices during the day, it becomes much easier to attain lucidity in dream and to then go on to other practices.

Often, and throughout the day, become vividly aware of exactly where you are and what you're experiencing in the moment. Wake up from the dream of distraction. The more often, the better. You don't need a special place or time—any place is good; any time is good. It only requires seconds for the moment of recognition, though it's good to increase the time as you are able.

It's particularly helpful to become aware as you react to situations. There's an immediate shift in the mind, allowing more flexibility to respond skillfully.

Make it a habit to turn awareness on itself, to try to be aware of awareness. Pay attention to what happens in that moment. Rest in that.

If you don't have immediate results, even if you practice for a long time before achieving lucidity in dream, don't be discouraged. Remember other skills it took time to develop, and how different your thoughts and behaviors are now relative to earlier times in your life. There is constant change. Knowing that nothing remains the same, you need not believe that how things manifest now will continue as they are.

The practice of lucidity during the day is as important as attaining lucidity at night. Experiencing the luminous, dreamlike qualities of life allows your experience to grow spacious, lighter, and more vivid. When lucidity is developed in dream and in waking, there is freedom to shape life positively, to finally give up the turmoil of being driven by hope and fear, desire and aversion. You can rest in presence.

CHAPTER 13

Preparation for the Night

Many of us carry the stress, emotions, thoughts, and confusions of the day into the night. There is no particular practice or time set aside to calm the mind and body before entering sleep. Instead, sleep comes in the midst of distraction, making it easy to remain connected to stress and worry throughout the night. When dreams arise from those states, there is little stability in presence. The dreamer is carried away by the images and interactions of the dream world. Sleep is disturbed. Dreams, if not stressful are, at best, merely a pleasant escape. Too often the sleeper wakes tired and unrested in the morning, often starting the day in an uneasy state.

Even for one who does not practice dream or sleep yoga, it is beneficial to prepare for sleep, to take it seriously. Calming the mind as much as possible before sleep, just as before meditating, generates stronger presence and positive qualities. Rather than carrying negative emotion into the night, use what skills you have to free yourself from such emotions. If you know how to allow emotion to self-liberate in emptiness, do so. If you know how to transform it or provide the antidote, then use that knowledge. Try to connect with the lama, *yidam*, and dakini; pray to the buddhas and deities; generate compassion, love, and gratitude. Do what you can to relax the tension in your body and let go of negative attitudes in your mind. Free of disturbance, with a light and easy mind, you will experience a more restful and healing sleep. Even if they are unable to do the rest of the practices, this is something positive everyone can incorporate into their daily lives.

Most spiritual traditions create sacred spaces and altars. They connect us to what they represent and change our inner state, affecting us as all environments do. You may not think of a bedroom as a sacred space, but when you practice dream and sleep yoga, it is. If you enter your bedroom as a place of contemplative practice, the environment will support positive mind states and emotions and your practice.

If the room is messy, straighten it up a bit, as you would a temple. Maybe place a small image of the dream goddess in your room. Put it near your bed to feel a stronger connection. Or use the image of another deity or buddha, your teacher, or another sacred image.

Small, inexpensive, battery-powered tea lights are easy to find online if not locally. If you have one, place it in front of the image or statue. When you look at the light, feel/imagine it connecting you to the goddess. Not the physical light but more the aftereffect, when you feel the light in you. That is the goddess, the luminosity of your mind's nature.

If it's not comfortable or practical to keep a light on all night, put a small, dim light by your bed (not a candle or anything with a flame). Look at it as you start to fall asleep, experience the luminosity for a short time, then shut it off before going to sleep.

Whatever you've done to make the environment supportive, consciously let it affect you as you fall asleep. Just remember the support is there, feel the luminosity and peace. The awareness of that luminosity will help to illuminate the darkness of your sleep.

The important point is to slow down before sleep, to listen to your body and be aware of what you are doing in your mind, how it is affecting you. Process the day. Let go of emotional disturbance. Relax your body and mind. Put your awareness in the central channel of the body. This enhances dreaming and lucidity.

Nine Purifications Breathing

You may have noticed how tension and stress in the body affects breathing. When someone with whom we are having difficulties walks into the room, the body tightens, and the breath becomes shorter and more constricted. When we are frightened, the breath comes quickly and is shallow. In sadness, breathing is often deep and punctuated by sighs. If someone we genuinely care for enters the room, we relax, and the breath opens and eases.

Rather than waiting for experience to alter the breath, we can deliberately use the breath to alter experience. The nine breaths of purification is a short practice to clear and purify the channels. The practice can be done before sessions of meditation, before sleep, and anytime you'd like to clear tensions and negativities from body and mind.

The practice is meant to purify the energies of the three poisons: ignorance, cleared through the central channel; anger and aversion, cleared through the white channel on the right; and attachment and desire, cleared through the red channel on the left.

The third foundational practice recommends reviewing the day before sleeping, remembering what occurred as a dream. It's helpful to do the review before the nine breaths practice, before getting into bed. Particularly note difficult emotions you felt during the day: anger; irritations; anxieties; frustrated attachments; disappointed hopes; moments of feeling lost and uncertain, dull or distracted. See them as elements of dream. These memories give you instances to use in the nine breaths practice, which you then begin.

The first three breaths are meant to clear negativities related to anger and aversion. Before you start the practice, bring to mind a specific situation or person toward which you feel anger, irritation, or aversion. It may be something you remembered during the review of the day. If not, use an earlier experience. Be specific. This isn't about abstract anger; it's *your* anger, irritation, harsh judgment. Recognize the emotion; it's likely to be something you feel frequently. It interferes, to a greater or lesser degree, with your flow of creativity, your sense of connection, your joy, and your loving relations with others. Give this review enough time that you feel the trace of the emotion in your body and mind. When you feel it, practice the first three breaths.

For the second three breaths, remember a recent experience of attachment, grasping, desire, or yearning. Remember it, feel it in your body, and take it into the practice.

For the third set of breaths, draw on a recent experience of ignorance. This is the fundamental poison—ignorance of the truth of oneself and the world. In personal situations, experiences arising from ignorance may manifest as uncertainty or confusion, a loss of purpose or direction, a lack of clarity, or numb indifference. Evoke the memory of an experience, feel it, then expel it with three exhalations through the central channel.

Nine Breaths Instructions

Sit in a cross-legged meditation posture or any comfortable posture with the back straight. Place the hands, palms up, in the lap, with the left hand resting on the right. Slightly draw in the chin to straighten the back of the neck. Take a moment to become present, aware, and relaxed.

Visualize the three primary channels. They are made of light. The central channel is blue. The right channel is white and the left is red.

First Three Breaths:
Clearing the White Channel of the Poison of Anger

Bring to mind a fresh experience of anger or aversion. Raise the right hand with the thumb pressing the base of the ring finger. Close the right nostril with the ring finger.

Slowly and deeply, inhale through the red left nostril, imagining the breath to be healing. Draw the breath down through the channel to the junction with the central channel, about four inches below the navel. Hold the breath there gently as you move the right ring finger to close the left nostril.

Exhale the breath through the white, right nostril, slowly and gently at first and more forcefully at the end to exhale completely.

Release your anger and aversion with each exhalation, letting it dissolve in space.

Traditionally you imagine releasing all obstacles linked with male potencies, anger and aversion, illness associated with the winds (prana), and obstacles and obscurations connected with the past. Let it all go. Repeat for three inhalations and three exhalations.

Second Three Breaths:
Clearing the Red Channel of the Poison of Attachment

Bring to mind a fresh experience of attachment. Maintaining openness in the white channel, change hands. Raise the left hand with the thumb pressing the base of the ring finger. Close the left nostril with the ring finger. Slowly and deeply inhale through the red channel, drawing the breath to the junction with the central channel. Hold the breath gently as you move your left hand to close the right nostril with the ring finger.

Exhale the breath through the left nostril, the red channel, slowly and gently at first and more forcefully at the end to exhale completely. With each exhalation, exhale the residue left by the experience you brought to mind. Exhale all obstacles linked with attachment and desire, with wanting things to be different than they are, and obstacles linked with female potencies and with illness associated with bile. Let go of all obstacles and obscurations connected with the future.

Repeat for three inhalations and exhalations. Feel openness in the white and red channels. Maintain the openness while you continue.

Third Three Breaths:
Clearing the Blue Channel of the Poison of Ignorance

Bring to mind a fresh experience of confusion, dullness, numbness, or distraction. Place the left hand on top of the right in the lap, palms up. Inhale deeply into both nostrils. Feel the breath move down the side channels to the juncture with the main channel, four finger widths below the navel. Hold the breath slightly before exhaling, gently in the beginning and forcefully enough to empty the lungs at the end. Visualize the exhalation rising up the central channel and out the top of the head, where it dissolves in clear space. Imagine, with each exhalation, expelling the felt residue of the memories you reviewed and expel potencies for illnesses associated with hostile spirits and with phlegm. Let go of all obstacles and obscurations associated with the present. Let go of all obstacles and obscurations arising from the ignorance of the samsaric mind. Feel the increasing openness of the blue central channel. Repeat for three inhalations and three exhalations.

Resting

Allow yourself to rest for as long as you like. Feel the openness of the channels. Feel the energies and tensions of mind and body calming. Be aware of freedom from anger, attachment, and ignorance. You may notice a sense of warmth as qualities of love, generosity, peace, and compassion arise. Rest in open awareness.

Guru Yoga

Guru yoga is an essential practice in all schools of Tibetan Buddhism and Bön. This is true in sutra, tantra, and Dzogchen. It develops the heart connection with the master. By continually strengthening our devotion, we come to the place of pure devotion in ourselves, the unshakable base of the practice. The essence of guru yoga is to merge the practitioner's mind with the mind of the master.

What is the true master? It is formless, the fundamental nature of mind, the primordial awareness at the base of all experience. Because we exist in dualism, it is helpful for us to visualize this inner guru as a form. Doing so makes skillful use of the conceptual mind, helping us stay directed toward practice and the generation of positive qualities.

In the Bön tradition, we often visualize Tapihritsa or the buddha Shenlha Ökar (gShen-Lha 'od-dKar) as the master. If you are already a practitioner, you may have another deity to visualize, such as Vajra Yogini, Guru Rinpoche, or a yidam. While it is important to work

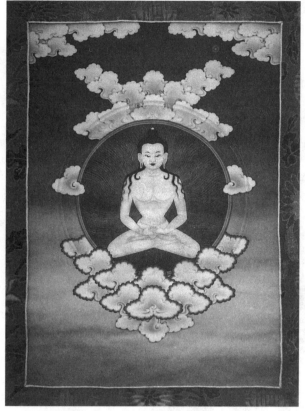

Tapihritsa

with a lineage with which you have a connection, understand that the master you visualize represents all masters with whom you are connected, your root teacher and all teachers with whom you have studied, and all·deities to whom you have commitments. The master in guru yoga is not an individual but the essence of enlightenment, the primordial awareness that is your own fundamental nature.

For dream yoga, it's helpful to visualize the dream goddess, Gyuma Chenmo, to make a connection with her. The dream goddess is not a concrete being. She is clarity and luminosity. Connecting with her supports us in realizing the goal of dream yoga She is protection as we enter sleep. She is the master, teacher, and guide. She is the nature of your own mind.

My teacher, Yongdzin Rinpoche, always emphasized the power of the tradition, the blessings that come down to us through an unbroken lineage stretching back many centuries. I recommend you connect to the source of this practice through guru yoga and prayer. Prayer focuses the mind and intention and connects us to the transmission of the lineage. You're not limited: pray to the dream goddess and other teachers and beings of refuge. Feel intense devotion, not to an image but to the living reality inside so intense that the tears may flow and your heart fills with love.

Let yourself merge with the guru's mind, your buddha-nature. This is how to practice guru yoga.

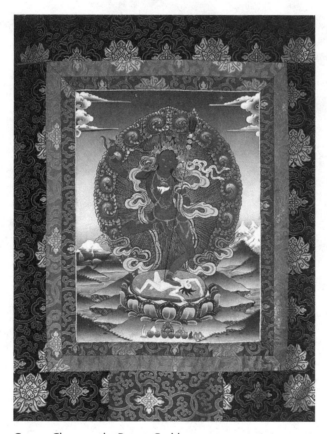

Gyuma Chenmo, the Dream Goddess

The Practice

After the nine breaths, still seated in meditation posture, visualize the master above and in front of you. Use your imagination to allow a being to exist there in three dimensions, made of light, pure, with a strong presence you can feel in your body, your energy, and your mind. Generate devotion and reflect on the great gift of the teachings and the good fortune you enjoy in having made a connection to them. Offer a sincere prayer, asking that your negativities and obscurations be removed, that your positive qualities develop, that you accomplish dream yoga.

Then imagine receiving blessings from the master in the form of three colored lights streaming from their three wisdom doors of body, speech, and mind. The lights should be transmitted in the following sequence: White light streams from the master's brow chakra into yours, purifying and relaxing your entire body and physical dimension. Then red light streams from the master's throat chakra into yours, purifying and calming your energetic dimension. Finally, blue light streams from the master's heart chakra into yours, purifying and quieting your mind.

When the lights enter your body, feel them. Suffused in wisdom light, use your imagination to make the blessing as real as possible. Let your body, energy, and mind rest. Let go of all tension. Let go.

After receiving the blessing, the master dissolves into light, enters your heart as light, and resides there as your innermost essence. Dissolve into the light in your heart center. Remain in pure awareness, rigpa.

There are more elaborate instructions for guru yoga involving prostrations, offerings, mudras, mantras, and more complicated visualizations. But the essence of the practice is merging your mind with the mind of the master, with pure awareness. Guru yoga can be done anytime during the day; the more often, the better. Many masters say that of all practices, guru yoga is the most important. It confers the blessings of the lineage, opens and softens the heart, and quiets the unruly mind. To completely accomplish guru yoga is to accomplish the path.

Protection

Going to sleep is a little like dying, a journey taken alone into the unknown. We completely lose ourselves in a void until, after some time, we arise again in a dream. When we do, we may have a different identity and a different body. We may be with people we do or don't know, experiencing a world unlike that of our waking lives.

Just trying to sleep in an unfamiliar place may occasion anxiety. Even if where we are is perfectly secure and comfortable, we do not sleep as well as we do at home in familiar surroundings. Maybe the energy of the place feels wrong. Or maybe it is only our insecurity disturbing us. Even in familiar places we may feel anxious while waiting for sleep to come or lying awake during the night, or we may be frightened by what we dream. When we fall asleep with stress, our dreams are mingled with fear and tension, sleep is less restful, and it's harder to stay engaged with the practice. So it is a good idea to create a sense of protection before we sleep and to turn our sleeping area into a sacred space.

This is done by imagining protective dakinis all around the sleeping area. Visualize the dakinis as goddesses, enlightened female beings who are loving, green in color, and powerfully protective. They remain near as you fall asleep and throughout the night, like mothers watching over a child or guardians surrounding a monarch. Imagine them everywhere, guarding the doors and the windows, sitting next to you, walking in the garden or the yard, and so on, until you feel completely protected. Use your imagination to make those protecting you as real as possible in your experience.

This may feel artificial, yet it doesn't feel artificial when we create anxiety, tension, or anger while dwelling on the dreamy memories of the past or worrying about imagined interactions and situations in the future. The quality of all experience is largely determined by the stories we tell in our minds. Using this faculty in practice is a positive use of imagination and has real benefit. Creating a protective, sacred environment in this way calms, relaxes, and promotes restful sleep.

This is how the mystic lives: seeing the magic; changing the environment and experience with the mind; recognizing that actions, including actions of the imagination, have significance.

The *Mother Tantra* tells us that as we prepare for sleep, we should maintain awareness of the causes of dreams, the object to focus on, the protectors, and ourselves. Hold these together in awareness not as many things but as a single environment. This will have a strong effect on dreaming and sleep.

This sounds like a lot to do before sleep, but it needn't be a burden. If you enjoy the practices and are not rushed, take as long as you like. If you're tired and need sleep, move through the practices quickly. The important point is to slow down for a while before going to bed. Relax, scan your body with awareness, progressively letting go of all tension from the top of your head to your feet. Clear your mind and infuse your heart with love and compassion. Enter sleep with gratitude for the chance to practice and generate strong intention to accomplish dream yoga.

Most important, if you don't have time to do the preparations, don't spend what time you do have doing the wrong things: worrying about the future, reliving or regretting the past, getting caught up in stressful thoughts.

CHAPTER 14

The Main Practice

To fully develop dream yoga, four tasks should be accomplished in sequence: (1) bringing awareness into the central channel; (2) cultivating clear vision and experience; (3) developing power and strength so we will not become lost; and (4) developing our wrathful aspect to overcome fear. In Tibetan iconography, deities are categorized by four related qualities: peaceful, joyful, powerful, and wrathful.

Although we may not feel connected to these positive qualities, they are in all of us, and we develop them further in dream yoga through the four main practices. They are assets in accomplishing the practice and benefit waking life.

In the first edition of this book, all four practices were to be done each night. The first before falling asleep, then waking every two hours to do the second practice, then the third, and finally the fourth. It's fine to practice this way if you like, especially if you are in retreat. But it's likely to disrupt sleep and negatively affect waking life. Instead, practice only one of the four steps for the entire night. If you wake during the night for any reason, bring your current practice to mind, touch on the visualization, generate the associated feeling, relax, and let yourself fall back into sleep.

This is how I teach the practice now, after almost thirty years of teaching dream yoga to many, many practitioners. This schedule is equally effective, if not more so, and far less disruptive.

The four steps are still to be done in sequence. Practice only the first step until you see results (this is explained later). Whether that takes weeks or months doesn't matter. Only then should you go on to the second practice and so on, obtaining results in the second practice before going on to the third, and in the third before going to the fourth. This will make the practice easier as you carry the results from one practice into the next. And it will be easier on your daily life.

If it works for you, schedule an intentional waking about two hours before your normal waking time. Research shows a large increase in lucid dreams after a waking period around that time. You've had most of the deep sleep you'll get for the night, and the dreams that follow are much longer, twenty minutes or even twice that.

While awake, try to recall the dreams you've had during the night, then repeat the preparation practices, with the exception of reviewing the day: pray, perform the nine breaths, practice guru yoga, and generate love and compassion throughout your body and mind. Most importantly, as much as possible during the waking period, strengthen the intention to be lucid in the coming dreams, repeating to yourself that you will recognize the dream as a dream with strong intent.

Try to remember something from a previous dream that you couldn't experience in waking life. It's particularly helpful if it's something you frequently encounter in a dream. With your imagination, rehearse recognizing the image in the next or in a future dream and using the recognition as a trigger to become aware that you are in a dream, to become lucid. Then return to the practice and fall asleep.

If it's hard to go back to sleep at this time, try waking up a half hour or an hour earlier the next morning. Sleep patterns are highly individual, and for some people, waking up earlier will make it easier to fall back to sleep.

When you have a lucid dream—when you are aware you are dreaming while you are dreaming—try to work with your dream. For example, if you are feeling fearful, change the fear to peacefulness. Try changing small to big, slow to fast. If you want to, fly, visit sacred places, or ask questions of the lineage masters. You can overcome any block, any limitation, because it is just a dream.

Chapter 20 provides instructions for the practices in outline form for easy reference. Read the following longer instructions first and return to them when needed to review details.

Bringing Awareness into the Central Channel

No matter how difficult the situation or how agitated, confused, or anxious we are, there is always peace deep inside. In this practice we connect to that peace by bringing awareness into the central channel. The key is in the throat chakra.

Lie on your right side with the knees bent enough to make the body stable. If it's comfortable, rest the left arm along your side and place the right hand under the cheek or pillow. We call this the lion posture.

Gentle the breath and relax the body. Allow the breathing to slow, to be full but so quiet that neither inhalation nor exhalation can be heard.

Visualize a beautiful four-petaled lotus made of deep red light, luminous, located in the throat chakra at the base of the throat. The chakra is closer to where the neck meets the shoulders than to the head. In the center of the four petals, facing forward, is an upright, luminous Tibetan *A*. It is clear, white, and translucent, like crystal made of light. The *A* represents your innate awareness, rigpa.

The energy of the throat chakra is sometimes a little strong, the energy of ego, of the demigods. It is represented by the red of the lotus as it colors the clear *A*. As the energy arises, visualize the white *A* on the red lotus and rest in clear awareness. Try to feel that luminous clarity.

Traditionally a crystal is laid on a red cloth as an illustration. The crystal seems to fill with and reflect red, even as it remains clear, transparent, and unstained. Similarly, as you practice, rest in the peaceful clarity and luminosity of pure awareness as experiences arise.

As you move toward sleep, relaxed and peaceful, lightly focus on the chakra, the red light, the clear *A*, and feel peace. Use your imagination to relax, to develop the experience of peace in your mind and throughout your body. As you merge with the luminous *A*, as you merge with peace, the mind rests in the central channel. This is the peace that is always available within. Connect to the feeling, become it, let go, sleep.

Don't use too much force. In the beginning, practitioners sometimes struggle, trying too hard and disrupting sleep. Don't fight with the practice. If you do, you'll lose the connection to peace. Instead, let the practice come to you: imagine, feel, merge with peace, fall asleep.

Visualization is easy for some, difficult for others. If visualization is difficult for you, it's not a problem. Feeling is more important than visualizing. Just imagine the *A* is there; you don't have to see it. Relax body and mind. Generate the feeling of peace throughout your body. Then become the peace. As you go to sleep, don't worry about losing focus on the *A*. If you do, you may go through the night struggling to connect, and that's not helpful. Instead, relax into peace, holding attention very lightly in the chakra. Gently let go into sleep. If you fall asleep feeling peace, this is good enough.

The teaching says focusing on this chakra produces gentle dreams. The example given is a dream in which a dakini invites the dreamer to accompany her. She helps the dreamer onto a mystical bird (garuda) or a lion and leads the dreamer to a pure land, a beautiful, sacred place. But this is cultural; the dream need not be this specific. Instead, you may walk in a garden or in the mountains, maybe guided by others, but the sign of success in the practice is the quality of peacefulness in the dream, whatever the imagery is.

Sometimes, when you connect to the slightly wrathful energy of the throat but lose your connection to awareness, disturbed dreams arise. This indicates a need to focus more on abiding in clear awareness, allowing experience of the red *A* to arise gently and peacefully, rather than being caught up in it.

As soon as you wake for any reason during the night, even for a moment, place your attention on the chakra and generate peace. If you sleep till morning, that's fine. Connect to peace as you wake.

Informal Practice

It's very helpful to practice informally during the day by bringing awareness into the central channel and connecting to inner peace. Repeat this again and again. When you're stuck in traffic, when you sit down at a desk or table or get into your car, when you have a still moment, return to the practice. Bring awareness to the throat. If you have time, bring your attention to the red lotus and the *A*. If not, just bring your attention to, and relax the base of the throat, and feel peace. This opens the chakra.

When the chakra is open, the quality of peace is available. Think of it this way: attention on the throat chakra opens the space there. The sense of space in the chakra is your awareness. The quality in the space is peace, which you can feel in the warm, red light. If you are, or once you become, familiar with inner peace, generate that experience as you do the practice, merging peace and awareness. Repeating this often during the day will support your practice at night. The result of the practice will manifest in waking life as well as in dreams as a stronger connection to peacefulness.

When you have results from the practice, when you can generate peace and find more peace in your waking life and in dreams, start the second practice.

Increasing Clarity

The second practice increases clarity. Clarity is the cognizant aspect of awareness, the luminosity of awareness allowing us to "see," to know what arises. By increasing clarity, we increase the vividness of awareness, of presence. The point of focus is the chakra located slightly above and behind where the eyebrows would meet on the brow. Visualize a white, luminous ball of light (*tiglé*) in the chakra.

It is a point of clarity. A tiglé, also known as *bindu*, can be many things and is translated in various ways. In one context, it is an energetic quality found in the body; in another, it represents unbound wholeness. As we use it in this practice, the tiglé is a small, luminous sphere of light. The different colored tiglés represent different qualities of consciousness. Visualizing them is meant to act as a door into the experience of that quality.

As in the first practice, take a comfortable position lying on your right side. A particular form of breathing is to be done. Inhale and hold the breath very gently. Lightly clench the perineum, the muscles of the pelvic floor, so you have the sense of pulling the held breath upward. Try to experience the breath as being held just below the navel, compressed by the pressure from below. It is difficult to imagine this kind of breathing; it may be necessary to experiment a bit until you discover the sense of it. Better yet is to receive detailed instruction from a teacher.

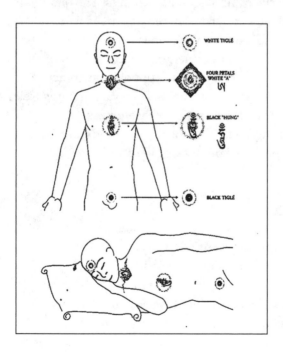

After holding the breath for a few moments, gently exhale. During the exhalation, relax the muscles in the pelvis, the chest, the whole body. Completely relax. Repeat this seven times.

Then allow yourself to fall asleep while resting in the luminosity, merging with it, lightly focused on the chakra. If you wake for any reason during the night, return your attention to the chakra.

The instruction to "visualize" the tiglé does not mean you should picture a static image of a round light. Instead, imagine yourself merging with luminosity in the chakra. Try to feel the tiglé with your imaginal senses and in your body, unifying completely with it until only clarity and luminosity exist. Some people will see the light with their internal visual sense, others will feel it more than see it. Feeling is more important than visualizing. Most important is to merge with the quality entirely.

When connected with the luminous tiglé in the brow chakra, the mind remains clear and present. As the experience of luminosity increases, becoming more vivid and spacious, allow yourself to be absorbed in the light of pure presence. If you sleep in this state, awareness is continuous through the night.

Developing clarity and continuity of awareness is the purpose of this section of the practice. This is what is meant by "increasing the luminosity of dream."

"Increasing" is what we call the quality of dreams manifested through this section of the practice. The sense here is of developing or growing toward completion, of generation, of bounty, of expansiveness and creativity. The example given in the *Mother Tantra* is of a dream in which a dakini plays musical instruments; sings; and brings flowers, fruit, and clothing to the dreamer. Again, this does not mean that the dreams must include a dakini or any other specific image, but as the practitioner strengthens in this part of the practice, the dreams will be characterized by enjoyment, creativity, and expansion.

The result manifests during the day as a sense of expansiveness and more vivid awareness of the present moment.

Informal Practice

When you have a few minutes during the day, bring your attention to the tiglé in the brow chakra. Not just to the external area—feel a sphere of light filling your head. Feel the light and spaciousness of awareness and the quality of it: the openness, the expansiveness, the clarity. Practice this as much as you like, particularly when you feel yourself tightening up and your vision becoming narrow. Connect with the luminosity of the mind, awareness open to whatever arises in it. Relax any tightness. Then return to what you were doing. Practicing this frequently will bring more openness in your waking experience and in dreams.

Strengthening Presence

When you experience results from the second practice and are ready, move on to the third practice. Again, it doesn't matter if this takes weeks or months. You have experience of inner peace from the first practice and clarity of awareness from the second. This is support for developing power, which in this context means developing presence, the strength to stay vividly aware without becoming lost in distraction. You can also return to earlier practices whenever you like, particularly if you feel the need to strengthen those qualities.

After the foundational practices during the day and preparatory practices before going to bed, you feel clean, clear. You've reviewed the day, recognized your memories as dream, and let them go. For this part of the practice, lie on your back, with your head, upper back, and shoulders on a high pillow. Cross the legs loosely, unlike in meditation posture; it doesn't matter which leg is on top. The position is somewhat similar to sleeping on a recliner; you recline but are not completely prone. Using a high pillow will help keep sleep light and generate more lucidity in dreams, but pay attention to the comfort of the neck. Do not remain in an uncomfortable position or disrupt your sleep.

It's important to pay attention to the needs of the body. When

I was a child, I sat cross-legged in school for many hours each day, so this position is very easy for me. But it is different for most Westerners. The idea is not to endure pain all night but to maintain continuity of awareness. Adjust the practice toward that goal.

Gently draw your attention to the heart area, the heart chakra. Inside the chakra is the black, luminous syllable HUNG. It faces forward just as the body does. Merge with the syllable so that everything is the black HUNG. Become the unconditioned awareness the HUNG represents. Let the mind be open and spacious, and rest lightly in the black HUNG.

The color black has to do with stability. It's the color associated with the changeless. It is strength. Rest your mind there and feel the space, the presence of the HUNG. Take twenty-one deep, gentle breaths, maintaining full awareness of breathing while the mind is merged with the black HUNG. Then let go and fall asleep.

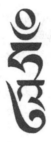

The Tibetan syllable HUNG

The quality being developed here is strength or power. You don't have to do anything; don't puff up or try to feel powerful. This is about finding the strength you already have inside. The sense of power is also one of security; dreams generated in this part of the practice have to do with the sense of secure power. The examples in the *Mother Tantra* are dreams in which a powerful dakini directs the dreamer to sit on a throne, the dreamer goes into a secure castle to receive teachings, or the dreamer is given approval by their father or mother. The quality is important, not the specific imagery. Instead of a dakini seating the dreamer on a throne, it may be someone celebrating the dreamer's accomplishments. Rather than a castle, the dream may take place in a situation that makes the dreamer feel secure, and instead of a parent, there may be another person in the dream who confers a sense of security, safety, and strength. The experience of being strongly in the present is the real result.

Informal Practice

As you did with the first two parts of the practice, bring your practice into your daily life. Several times during the day, focus on your heart area. Your attention is clear, and you're not thinking of something else. Your awareness is open, not tight. It rests in the area of your heart. You can think of it this way: you draw your attention to the heart chakra and feel the silence there, feel the spaciousness there. This is the silence and spaciousness of your awareness when it is undistracted.

In that clear, open awareness, visualize/imagine the black HUNG in the heart center. Feel the stability and strength of it, the power of being. This is your inner strength. It emerges from stability in the clarity of awareness. Recognize the quality and stay connected to the strength. Sit longer. If you get lost, let go of distraction. Return to the HUNG and abide in clear awareness. Stay connected.

As you do this again and again, you naturally become familiar with the experience of stability in strong presence. The symbol becomes a way to connect to it. As you develop this awareness during the day, you will start to find the quality of power in dreams. Practicing day and night, you will take the strength of presence into your thoughts, your emotional experience, your relationships and work, and your meditation practice.

This is the template for the informal practices of all four sections of the main practice. Strengthening the connection to a quality, being able to generate the felt sense of the quality in dreaming and waking, and using the generation of the qualities to develop the continuity of the practice through the entire cycle of day and night—peace, vivid awareness, stable presence, fearlessness.

Developing Fearlessness

In the fourth part of the dream yoga practice there is no particular position to take; just make yourself comfortable. There is no pre-scribed breathing; the breath is left in its natural rhythm.

The "secret chakra," the chakra behind the genitals, is the point of focus. Inside the chakra is a black tiglé—a sphere of black, luminous light. This is the darker aspect of the imagination. The teaching says dreams generated here are likely to contain wrathful dakinis, fire on the mountain and in the valley, torrential rivers, and winds destroying everything in their path. These are dreams in which the elements destroy the images of the self. The dreams can be terri-fying; discover if this is true for you. The quality of dreams in this section of the night may eventually become wrathful, providing the opportunity to develop fearlessness.

In practice, you enter the black, luminous tiglé in the secret chakra and become it. Then let your mind relax and just lightly focus on the luminous black light that is everywhere, pervading your senses and mind, and allow yourself to sleep.

The four qualities—peaceful, joyful, powerful, and wrathful—are broad bands of associated images, feelings, emotions, and expe-riences. It is not necessary to have the specific kinds of dreams presented as examples in the teachings. It is the quality that is important, the emotional timbre, the felt sense of the dream. This is how to determine to which chakra the dream is connected, to which dimension of experience; it is not done by trying to decipher the dream contents.

Informal Practice

As before, when you have a few minutes during the day, let the mind return to the black tiglé. What does fearlessness feel like? It isn't aggressive or reckless; it's stability in awareness. Just as you can be challenged in wrathful dreams, you can use moments of fear, worry, or anxiety during the day as reminders and opportunities to return to the practice. Instead of getting caught up in uneasy thoughts, immediately let them go by putting your attention in the black tiglé. Relax the body and breath, and feel the space there, the openness. When you do, the quality of fearlessness arises. Become familiar with the process; develop the quality until fearlessness becomes stable.

Return to the practice if you wake during the night. When you awake in the morning, be aware of waking and stay present. Develop continuity of awareness through the night, across the periods of sleeping and waking, and during the whole day.

Integrating the Practice

This section gives more detail on integrating the practice during waking hours. It refers to the third practice but is an example of how to work with all four practices.

The third principal practice is meant to strengthen presence. How can you apply the practice in everyday life?

Most of us have the experience of being in situations where we feel secure in ourselves. We are confident and comfortable, able to respond intentionally to what is happening. We remain aware and flow with experience rather than struggle with it.

We probably also know the unpleasant sense of being unstable in ourselves, at a loss regarding how to respond to a situation. This inner instability has much to do with losing the ability to remain stable in awareness of the present moment. Instead, we are dragged into turbulent thoughts and emotions, become tense or uncomfortable in our bodies, and respond to the narratives playing out in the imagination rather than to what is actually unfolding.

Strengthening presence, staying connected to clear awareness in the present moment, is the source of the power to remain undistracted by the stories running through the mind. When we aren't pulled away from the moment, we have the capacity to respond wisely and positively.

To apply the practice in waking life, start by asking yourself where and when you feel a lack of presence, of being unable to stay centered. You may feel insecure in relationships, vulnerable and uncertain. You may be comfortable in relationships but feel weak in work settings. In social settings, you may withdraw or take on a social identity to hide behind.

Take some time to reflect on this. Recognizing the situations or relationships in which you feel this disconnection from your deeper self is helpful. It supports your practice. When you find yourself in a situation that is likely to cause this disconnection, you can appreciate it as an opportunity to practice. You needn't wait for a dream at night; the dream is unfolding during the day.

You are there in the situation. You feel the familiar instability, uncertainty, anxiety, irritation, fragmentation, or distraction and *immediately* recognize an opportunity to practice. Draw clear, open attention to your heart area. Feel the HUNG in the center of the chakra. Feel the space in your heart open and expand. Remain in the present, in awareness. If you get lost, let go of the distraction and become present again. Choose to respond positively, even if the response is only in your mind. Open, accept, stay present.

What if you don't feel strength and don't remain present? That's okay. Just keep returning to the practice. Familiarize yourself with abiding in open awareness, using the heart as an anchor, even if only for a moment. Importantly, notice those moments and how the transition from distraction to presence feels: how the mind and heart open, how it is different from the experience of being lost in the stories in your mind. The strength will come as you practice, eventually manifesting as a quiet security. Paying attention to the change enhances the experience.

Beyond noticing the change, try to abide in awareness for longer periods. If you spend five minutes practicing and working to draw clear, open attention to your heart, you may begin to feel a change. You are aware of the quality arising as you stabilize in open awareness. You feel the difference. Recognizing the difference, expand the experience, prolong it, cultivate familiarity. We call this *gom*. It is important, so continue for the next five minutes, ten minutes, however long you have for practice. Over time, situations that once led to distracted uncertainty and turmoil now become signals to turn to the practice of presence.

Use this method to develop the peace of the first practice, the luminosity of the second, the power of the third, and the fearlessness of the fourth. This is integrating the practice into daily life. But the practice itself goes much deeper. Abiding in clear, vivid awareness is the essence of the path.

More on the Elements of the Practice
Sequence

Each section of the practice evokes a particular energetic quality of consciousness to be integrated with awareness, and each quality supports the development of the next. Because of this development, the four sessions are practiced in order.

The first part of the practice is imbued with the peaceful aspect of dreams. It's much easier to work with this aspect than, for example, the wrathful one. It is easier to stay present in a peaceful situation than a frightening one. It is a general principle of practice to work more frequently with situations that are easier to master and practice with more difficult situations as we develop. In this case, we first develop focus and stability in peace and then work with more challenging aspects of experience.

The first practice is not so much about trying to develop something as it is about rediscovering restful awareness. There is less trying to do and more allowing to be. It is as if, after running around all day, you come home and relax into peaceful dreams. It takes a bit of time to rest up and be restored. The chakra used is the throat chakra, which is energetically connected to inner peace.

When you move to the second practice, increasing clarity, you bring with you the access to peace, and this changes the attitude and quality of the mind. Cultivating peace and stability in the first practice is like establishing a base in the body. In the second session, you ornament the body by developing a vivid, luminous awareness.

Therefore, the focus is on the chakra behind the brow, which is connected with opening and increasing clarity.

If stability is developed in the first session and clarity in the second, then power can be developed in the third. The focal point is the most central chakra in the body, the heart chakra, which is connected to the source of strength. The power cultivated here is the power over thoughts and the power to be free of habitual reactivity when encountering appearances. Like a ruler sitting on a throne—the seat of power—you sit in the base of your power, in pure awareness.

In the fourth part of the night—based on stability, clarity, and power—fearlessness is developed. We have within us the causes for frightening dreams. After some accomplishment in the first three stages of the practice, we call them out by focusing on the black tiglé in the secret chakra, the chakra most closely connected to wrathful karmic traces. The generation of frightening dreams is, here, a result of practice, and the practitioner is encouraged to continue dreams of this kind, to use the practice to transform even frightening karmic traces into the path. In this way, we test our development in the practice and further strengthen the qualities we have cultivated. Frightening images and situations in dreams are welcomed as opportunities for developing the practice. In the same way, we use difficult situations in waking moments to develop stability in awareness.

Position

Where I come from, most people sleep on a three-by-six-foot Tibetan carpet. If you move around too much, you fall out of bed. That does not usually happen, because when you sleep on something small, the position of the body is held in the sleeping mind throughout the night. If you sleep on a narrow ledge, it's natural to maintain enough awareness to keep from rolling off the edge. Here, in the big beds of the West, a sleeper can rotate like the hands of a clock and not fall out, but holding one position will help maintain awareness.

You can experiment with this when you find your concentration scattered. Change your position, straighten your back and neck and calm and gentle the breath; you may find you can concentrate quite well. Breathing, the movement of prana, the position of the body, thoughts, and the quality of mind are all interrelated. Unfolding this understanding allows the practitioner to consciously generate positive experiences.

The postures recommended in the tradition can be disruptive if you're not used to them. They are meant to help align the energy body with the practice. If the postures are comfortable for you, good. If not, let them go. Discomfort is not support; it's an obstacle. Just practice with the symbols and locations. For example, in the first practice, visualize the lotus and the red *A* in the throat chakra while maintaining a comfortable posture. Your goal is to merge with the quality, in this case, peace; not to focus on discomfort.

Focusing the Mind

Just as various body postures alter the flow of energy and affect the quality of experience, so do different visualizations focused in the body. Each of the four parts of the main practice involve focusing on a tiglé or syllable in one of four chakras.

Those focus points are not really there. The object of visualization is like a drawing or symbol representing patterns and qualities of energy that move through that location. By using these images, the mind is better able to connect to the particular patterns of energy where they are concentrated most strongly. Color also has an effect in consciousness, as we know from daily experience. If we enter a room painted red, our experience is quite different than it would be if we entered a white room, a green room, or a black room. Color is used in visualization to help establish a quality in consciousness.

To experience how the visualizations affect consciousness, try this: imagine being in total darkness, complete blackness. Not only is it dark around you, but it is dark in your vision, on your skin, above and below you, inside every cell of your body. Sounds continue but in complete darkness. It is almost as if you can feel, smell, and taste the darkness.

Now imagine the darkness suddenly giving way to clear, pervasive light—around you, in you, light that is you. If you play with this, you may be able to feel the difference in the two visualizations through the subtle imaginal senses that illuminate your internal world, not just the visual aspect of the imagination. In the dark, you have one experience, perhaps even a little fear; in the light, there is clarity.

Here is another experiment meant to give you experience of the kind of focus the practice requires. Relax your body. Imagine a red, luminous *A* in your throat chakra. The red light is deep, rich, and sensuous. Use your imagination to feel the light. Let it calm you, relax you, quiet your mind and body, heal you. The light expands, filling your throat chakra, then your entire body. As it does, it relaxes every tension. Everything it touches dissolves into red light. Your entire body dissolves into red light. Let the light pervade your awareness so that all you see is luminous red light; all you feel is calm red light; any sound you hear is peaceful red light. Do not think this through—experience it. Let your mind be red light so there is no "you" being aware of an object, only the red light being awareness itself. Allow whatever arises as subject or object to dissolve into red light. Everything—body and energy, world and mental events— dissolves until you are completely merged with red light. There is no "inside" or "outside," only red light. This is how to merge with the *A* and how to focus at night, unified with the experience behind the visualization.

As meditators we sometimes think of concentration as a switch that is either on or off, but this is not the case. Awareness can be focused in varying degrees of intensity. For example, when I came out of a long dark retreat, all visual phenomena were extremely intense. The houses and the trees, every color and every object, were vibrant. When I saw these same images day after day, they were unremarkable, but after fifty days of total darkness, my focus on vision was so strong that everything was extraordinarily vivid. As the days went by, the visual phenomena seemed to dim, but of course the phenomena had not changed—it was my awareness of them that had diminished. Although the circumstances of my experience were unusual, they illustrate a general principle. All of our experiences will be more vivid if we focus on the present without distraction.

In the practice there are gradations in the intensity of focus. When just beginning the visualization at night, there may be a very strong focus on the tiglé. As the body relaxes and sleep comes, the appearance of the visualization weakens. The senses fade, and there is less hearing, smelling, touching, and so on. The awareness diminishes in intensity and acuity. Next, there may be almost no feeling, another level of focus. Finally, there is no sensory experience at all and no image of the visualization.

It's likely you have naturally experienced maintaining a focus throughout the night; for example, when you need to wake for an early appointment, some awareness remains during sleep. Let's say you have to get up at five in the morning. You go to sleep but keep waking to check the clock. The awareness of the need to wake early remains, although you are not strongly conceptualizing it, not thinking about it. The focus is subtle. This is the kind of focus to bring to the practice—not strong concentration but a light touch, gentle yet consistent. If you are joyful before falling asleep because something wonderful happened in your life, each time you wake, you wake to joy. It is continuous through sleep; you need not hang on to it. Your awareness simply rests with it. This is the way to be with the tiglé: sleep with it as you sleep with joy.

Two relationships to phenomena are relevant to focusing on the tiglé. In one, phenomena are grasped by the mind. In the other, phenomena appear to the mind. Grasping is a grosser form of dualistic interaction. The object is treated as a separate, distinct object—and the mind holds on to it. When grasping ceases, it does not mean dualism is gone—phenomena still arise in experience and are conceptualized as separate entities—but the conceptualization is subtler. It might be said that the first is a more aggressive, active conceptualization, while the second is more passive, simply allowing phenomena to appear in awareness. As it is weaker, it is easier to dissolve in pure awareness.

We begin the practice with the grosser form. Conceptualize the object and develop as strong an experience of it as possible using the imaginal senses. Try to visualize it clearly and, more importantly, feel it and let it affect the sensations in the body and the quality of the mind. After strongly establishing the object in awareness, loosen the grip. Let the object appear without effort as if intention, lying below the surface of consciousness, binds the mind to the object. Just as the mind stays connected to the need to wake for an early appointment or to a great joy, there is no need for exertion or concentration—the object just appears, and you are with it. You are no longer creating it; you are allowing it, observing it. It is similar to lying in the warm sun with your eyes closed. Without concentrating on the sun being "out there," you are warm, with the light, not separate from it. You do not have an experience of warmth and light—you need not try to keep your concentration on them—your experience *is* warmth and light; you are merged with them. This is how to be with the visualization during practice.

One common problem encountered in the beginning of practice is the disruption of sleep that occurs when the focus is held too tightly. The focus should be light, without force. The parallel to this in ordinary sleep is the difference between having images and thoughts drift through the mind as you fall asleep and being emotionally and intensely fixed on thoughts and memories, which leads to insomnia.

Let experience teach you. Pay attention to what works and what doesn't, and adjust. If the practice keeps you awake, incrementally reduce the intensity of the focus until you can sleep.

Focusing on the tiglé or syllable, whether by grasping or by letting it appear, is a first step. The real intent is to become unified with the experience the object symbolizes. As an example, the letter *A* is the symbol of the unborn, unchanging, natural state of mind. Rather than focusing on it as an object, it is best to merge with the pervasive awareness it represents. Awareness can be cultivated in sleep because it is already there.

Beyond letting the object appear to the mind, there is nondual presence. The image may or may not remain, but in either case, experience is not divided into subject and object. There is only awareness, and you are it. This is the significance of the clear *A* being tinged red by the color of the lotus petals. Our innate awareness is symbolized by the *A*. When experience arises as symbolized by the red of the petals, it colors the *A*, but the luminosity of rigpa is not lost.

Often practitioners say they have a hard time maintaining the visualization or that the visualization interferes with sleep. The progression is to see it, feel it, and then be it. As you merge with the object, the visualization may cease. This is not a problem. To sleep, you have to let go.

The teaching also prescribes this kind of focus at the time of death. Maintaining this presence is the essence of the practice of the transference of consciousness at the time of death (*phowa*). In this practice, the intention is to move the mind directly into the pure space of awareness (dharmakaya). If successful, the practitioner does not experience the turbulence and distraction of the after-death experience but instead is liberated directly into the clear light.

Without the ability to remain in pure presence, we are distracted and wander off into dreams, fantasies, samsara, the next life. If we abide in pure presence, we find ourselves in the clear light during the night, remain in the nature of mind during the day, and are liberated in the bardo after death.

CHAPTER 15

Lucidity

If someone tells us they spent many years in retreat, we are impressed and rightly so; this kind of effort is needed to attain enlightenment. But in our busy lives, such a thing may seem to be impossible. We may wish to do a traditional three-year retreat, but our circumstances will never allow it.

Actually, we all have the possibility of doing this much practice. During the next ten years of life, we will spend three years in sleep. Maybe we simply ignore dreams. But if we remember them, even pieces of them, we may have lovely experiences. We may also practice anger, jealousy, or fear. Perhaps these are emotional experiences we need to have, but we do not need to continue in such a way that we increase the habitual inclination to be attached to and driven by emotions and fantasies. Why not practice the path instead? Those three years of sleep can be spent in practice. Once lucidity is stabilized, any practice can be done in dream—some more effectively and with more consequence than when practiced in the day.

Dream yoga develops the capacity we all have for lucid dreaming. A lucid dream, in this context, is one in which the dreamer is aware during the dream that they are dreaming. The majority of people have had at least one experience of lucid dreaming, and it's common in childhood. It may have been in a nightmare in which we realized we were in a dream and woke to escape. Or it may just have been an unusual experience we still remember. Some people regularly have lucid dreams without any intention of doing so, but most of us do not. As the preliminary and main practices are integrated into the life of the practitioner, lucid dreams will begin to occur with increasing frequency. Lucid dreaming is not in itself the goal of practice, but it is an important development along the path of this yoga.

There are different levels of lucid dreaming. At the superficial level, you may realize you're in a dream but have little clarity and no power to affect the dream. Lucidity is found and then lost. At the other end of the continuum, lucid dreams can be extraordinarily vivid, feeling "realer" than ordinary waking experience.

As you practice the foundational practices during the day, you develop a greater continuity of awareness, a greater lucidity, and you become freer to choose how to respond to experience. You practice by guiding your thoughts, speech, and behavior to shape situations and inner experience in a positive direction. As you do, you practice developing stability in clear awareness.

The same is true in dream. If you are lucid in a dream, you have freedom. You can then practice by transforming yourself and the dream until the boundaries and limitations of the mind and identity are overcome. Then you can literally do anything you can think of to do. The mind becomes flexible.

Why is flexibility of mind so important?

Wrong views and the rigidities arising from desire and aversion keep us trapped in the mind's stories and delusions. Different people sharing the same situation react differently. Some grasp more, and some less. The more grasping there is—the more reacting from karmic conditioning—the less freedom. Instead we are controlled by the experiences we encounter.

Flexibility of mind is the capacity that, when developed, allows us to let go of habitual reactions. We can then choose to lessen grasping and aversion and abide in clear awareness. We can accept things as they are and respond positively to what occurs. Like a mirror, we can welcome whatever arises. We lack this flexibility now because we do not understand that what appears in awareness, and our reactions to it, is the reflection of our own minds. As we practice transformation in dream and our daily life, we are able to experience the truth of this directly.

In lucid dreams, we practice transforming what is encountered. As we break habitual limitations of experience, the mind becomes supple and calm. We are less inhibited by our constructed identities when we have the experience of transforming them and letting them go in dreams. We are less constricted by our habitual perceptions when we have experience of how subjective they are. The purpose of these practices is to integrate lucidity and flexibility with every moment of life, to let go of the heavily conditioned way we have of ordering reality and of making meaning. To wake from delusions.

Developing Flexibility

The teachings suggest many things to do in dreams after lucidity has been developed. The first step in developing flexibility in dream, as in waking, is to recognize the potential for doing so. As we think about the possibilities suggested in the teachings, the mind incorporates them into its potential. We become capable of having experiences we could not imagine before.

If I click on one of the icons on the screen of my computer, a file opens. Click on another, and something else appears on the screen. The mind is like that. The attention goes to something, and like clicking on an icon, suddenly a train of thought and images appear. The mind keeps clicking, moving from one thing to another. Sometimes we have two windows open, as when we are talking to someone and also thinking about something else. Ordinarily we don't think of this as having multiple selves or multiple identities, but we can manifest those multiple selves in a dream. Rather than simply having our attention divided, in dream we can divide into different, simultaneously existing dream bodies.

One night, after working on the computer, I dreamt I was looking at a screen on which icons would appear. I could click on them with my mind, changing the whole environment. An icon for forest appeared, and when I clicked on it, I was in a forest. Then an icon for ocean popped up, and after clicking on it, I was suddenly in an ocean setting. The capacity to do this was in my mind, but the specific experience arose after the interaction with my computer. Thoughts influence subsequent thoughts.

Dream practice works with this. The teachings present us with new ideas, new possibilities, and the tools to realize them. Then it's up to us to manifest those possibilities in dreams and waking life.

For instance, the teachings talk about multiplying things in dream. Perhaps we dream of three flowers. Because we are aware of being in a dream and the flexibility of dream, we can make a hundred flowers, a thousand flowers, a rain of flowers. But first we need to recognize the possibility. If we do not know this multiplication of objects is an option, then, for us, the option does not exist.

Research with dreams in the West has found that people can improve skills by practicing them in dreams and daydreams. Centuries ago, this understanding was incorporated in the teachings. This need not be directed only to skills to aid us in daily life; it can be applied at the most profound levels of spiritual life. Practicing transformation in dream is the same as tantric practices in which you transform yourself. It has the same goals and benefits, but it is much easier to accomplish in a dream because you actually transform.

Always aim for the highest, most inclusive goal, as this will automatically take care of the lesser. While it is good to work on relative issues, after enlightenment, there are no problems at all.

The *Mother Tantra* lists eleven categories of experience in which the mind is usually bound by appearance. All of these are to be recognized, challenged, and transformed. The principle is the same in all of them, but it's helpful to spend time thinking about each to introduce the possibilities of transformation to your mind. The categories are size, quantity, quality, speed, accomplishment, transformation, emanation, journey, seeing, encounter, and experience.

Size. Change your size in a dream, becoming as small as an insect and then as large as a mountain. Take a big problem and make it small. Take a small flower and make it as large as the sun or hold the moon in your hand.

Quantity. If there is one buddha in your dream, increase the number to one hundred or one thousand. If there are one thousand problems, make them one. In dream practice, you can burn the seeds of incipient karma. Using awareness, drive the dream rather than be driven; dream rather than let yourself be dreamt.

Quality. When people get stuck in an unwholesome experience, it is often because they don't know it can be changed. Think about the possibility of change and then practice it in a dream. When you are angry in a dream, change that emotion to love. You can change the qualities of fear, jealousy, anger, greed, and dullness. None of these are helpful. Tell yourself they can be overcome by transforming them. You can even say this out loud to strengthen your knowing. This is the practice when awake too. It's easier in a dream, but it's not meant to be practiced only in dreams. Once you have the experience, do the same in waking life and vice versa— practice this in waking life, and it becomes easier in dream. This develops freedom and flexibility. You do not need to remain trapped by prior conditioning.

Speed. In just a few seconds of dream, many things can be accomplished because you are entirely in the mind. Slow down an experience until each moment is a whole world. Visit a hundred places in a minute. The only boundaries in a dream are boundaries in imagination.

Accomplishment. Whatever you have been unable to accomplish in life, you can accomplish in dreams. Do practices, write a poem, travel to another planet. Speak to a crowd of a thousand if you are afraid of public speaking, walk a tightrope across a deep canyon if you're afraid of heights, finish what needs finishing.

A year after my mother passed away, she appeared in my dream and asked for help. I asked her what I could do. She gave me a drawing of a stupa and asked that I build it for her. I knew I was dreaming, but I accepted the task as if it were real. I was in Italy at the time, where there are many building restrictions and zoning laws. I did not know how to get the permits, the money, or the land I needed. So I thought to ask my guardians. This is what the *Mother Tantra* recommends: ask the dream guardians for help when confronted with a task that it seems you cannot accomplish.

In response to my request for help, the guardians appeared. A giant bodhi tree stood in the dream, and suddenly the guardians turned it into the stupa. In our culture, we believe that building a stupa for someone who has died helps that person to go on to their next birth. My mother was happy and satisfied in the dream, and so was I. I felt I had given her something important, something that had not happened at home in India when she died. Now it was accomplished, and my mother and I were both happy. The feeling carried over into my waking life.

The accomplishments in dream influence waking life. By working with experience, you work with the karmic traces. Use the dream to accomplish what is important to you.

Transformation. Transformation is very important for practitioners of tantra as it is the principle underlying tantric practice. But it is also important for all of us. Learn to transform yourself. Try everything. Transform into a bird, a dog, a garuda, a lion, a dragon. Transform from an angry person into a compassionate person, from a grasping, jealous human into an open, clear buddha. Transform yourself into the yidam and the dakini. This is very powerful for developing flexibility and overcoming the limitations of habitual identities.

Emanation. This is similar to transformation. After transforming yourself into a yidam or a buddha, emanate many more bodies that can be of benefit to other beings. Duplicate yourself and be in two bodies, then three, four, as many as you can, and then more. Break through the limitation of experiencing yourself as a single, separate ego.

Journey. Start with places you wish to go. You want to go to Tibet? Take a trip there. To Paris? Where have you always wanted to go? Where have you been afraid to go? Go!

This is not simply arriving somewhere; this is about the journey. Guide yourself there consciously. You can travel to another country, to a pure land where there is no defilement, or to a place you have not seen in many years. Almost every night I go back to India—a cheap way to travel. Visit the bottom of the ocean or the center of the earth, fly to the moon. Loosen the constrictions binding your mind.

Seeing. Try to see what you have not seen before. Have you ever seen Guru Rinpoche? Tapihritsa? Christ? Now you can. Have you seen Shambhala or the center of the sun? Have you seen cells dividing in your body or your heart pumping or the top of Mount Everest or the view from a bee's eye? Generate ideas for yourself and then make them real in dreams.

Encounter. In the Tibetan traditions, we have many stories of people meeting teachers, guardians, dakinis, and so on in their dreams. Maybe you feel a connection to teachers of the past or present; now you can meet them. When you do, ask right away if you can meet a second time. That creates more of an opportunity to meet again. Then ask for teachings.

Experience. Use a dream to experience something you have not done yet. If you are uncertain about your experience of rigpa, have it in the dream. Do you want to feel the prana move in the channels and chakras? Experience that. You can experience any mystic state or stage of the path, however elaborate or simple. You can breathe underwater like a fish, walk through walls, or become a cloud. You can travel the universe as a beam of light or fall as rain from the sky. Whatever you can think of, you can do.

The principle of developing flexibility in dream is more important than the particulars, just as the luminous quality of the crystal is more important than the color of light it happens to be reflecting. Suggestions from the teachings should not become more limits. Go beyond them. Think up new possibilities and manifest them until whatever seems to limit your experience is directly experienced as fragile and nonbinding. If conditioned by the apparently solid entities we encounter, they can be transformed in our experience, made luminous and transparent. As we are conditioned by the apparent solidity of thoughts, they can be dissolved in the limitless freedom of the mind. Work at the boundaries of experience, the constrictions of conditioning and limiting beliefs. Your identity is more flexible than you can imagine.

There is a basic principle for the spiritual journey that we should continue to exercise even in the freedom of the dream. The possibilities in dream are unlimited, and we can make whatever changes to the dream we wish, but it is important to change toward the positive. This best serves our spiritual path. Actions taken in dream have an effect on us internally and condition our future just as actions taken in waking life do. There is tremendous freedom in dream, but there is no freedom from karmic cause and effect. We need patience and strong intention to develop the flexibility necessary to overthrow the dictates of negative conditioning.

Treat your dreams with respect and incorporate all experiences of dream, like your waking life, into the path. Lucidity brings more light to the mind; exercising flexibility undoes the conditioning that constricts it. Using a dream to develop freedom from limitations, to overcome obstacles in your path, and finally to recognize your true nature and the true nature of all phenomena is to use the dream wisely.

CHAPTER 16

The Obstacles

The *Mother Tantra* describes four obstacles that may be encountered in dream yoga: distraction in delusive fantasy, laxity, restlessness that results in waking, and forgetting. It prescribes internal and external remedies.

Delusion and Losing Yourself

It's easy to get lost in the mind's stories during the waking state. Even if we try to remain consciously aware of the moment, the situations in life and our conditioning are such that almost anything can capture our attention and carry it away. Something appears in the mind—an interaction with someone, something we've seen or heard, a thought of the future or a memory—and we are lost in stories, emotions, judgments, plans, and reactions. We are caught up in the dream of the day and lose connection to clear awareness.

In the dream of night, it's the same. As soon as the dream arises, you're lost in the content, in reacting to what appears to be real. You don't recognize that it's "only a dream." The Ma Gyu calls this the obstacle of delusion. Delusion because we are caught up by, and chase after, appearances that do not exist in the way we think they do. They are only in the mind, reflections of the mind. They are not real in themselves.

The internal antidote is to focus on the central channel. What does this feel like? Try it; you'll find you feel centered and present, you come out of fantasy and back to yourself, to the present moment. It is helpful to fall asleep with awareness in the central channel. Be simple in this. Just feel the central channel, put your attention there. This will prevent the mind from running away.

The Ma Gyud recommends meditating on impermanence and the illusory nature of dualistic experience. When we take the contents of dream to be real and solid, we are caught up in the story and become lost. Recognizing appearances as insubstantial and temporary makes it easier to remain undistracted, allowing us to abide in clear awareness.

The external antidote is to make an offering or do devotional practices like guru yoga. Dream yoga is not just psychological; it's a spiritual practice. Trust in teachers and teachings, in enlightened beings, in the dream goddess. The ability to open your heart and pray affects the results of the practice positively. If your goal is only to have lucid dreams, this doesn't matter. But if your goal is higher illumination, then it is helpful to make these connections.

Laxity

The second obstacle is laxity. It manifests as an internal laziness, a lack of internal strength and clarity. When you are lax in practice, you may be comfortable but your attention is weak. You are not fully present even while attending to the object of focus. This is different than the first obstacle, in which your attention chases a distraction. In this case the mind is dull or clouded.

The antidote is to visualize blue smoke slowly drifting up the central channel from the junction of the three channels (a few inches below the navel and in the center of the body) to the throat. Don't get distracted by thinking of where the smoke goes, if it collects, and that kind of thing. Just visualize the smoke slowly moving up the central channel, as if already in a dream.

The *Mother Tantra* suggests that when laxity occurs, you may be encountering a problem with a spirit or with a force in your environment. A Tibetan may then visit a teacher or healer to ask for something like an exorcism.

Self-Distraction

The third obstacle is self-distraction. You wake again and again and are restless in sleep. This may be a problem with prana, or you may be excited or agitated. The antidote is to focus on the four petals of a lotus in the throat chakra. On each is a dakini represented by a tiglé. The tiglé to the front of your body is yellow. The one on your left is green. To your back is the red tiglé, and to your right is the blue. If there is a problem with restless self-distraction, focus on the tiglés one after the other as you fall asleep. Try to feel protector dakinis in all directions.

Externally, doing the chöd practice, a ritual offering to spirits, can be of benefit. Also determine if you have broken commitments (*samaya*) you made involving the teaching or your teachers. Disturbed relationships with friends may also cause this restlessness.

Self-confession can be useful. To do this, visualize your teacher or your objects of refuge, as in guru yoga, and confess what is wrong. Examine it, not with guilt or shame but with awareness. If you did something that was not right, decide not to do it again. Perhaps there is an action that should be taken, such as talking with the friend with whom you are disturbed. If so, you can decide to take such an action.

Forgetting

The fourth obstacle is forgetting—forgetting your dreams and forgetting to practice. Even if you have helpful experiences, they may be forgotten. A personal retreat can bring more clarity to the mind. Balancing the prana using the breath can settle and steady the awareness. The *Mother Tantra* prescribes the first primary practice, the practice focusing on the *A* at the throat, as an antidote. Keep awareness on the *A* while falling asleep. This will help you remember. As soon as you wake, record even snippets of dreams. This will create the habit of turning to your dream in the moment of awakening.

Four Obstacles according to Shardza Rinpoche

Shardza Rinpoche also writes of four possible obstacles but categorizes them differently: problems with prana, mind, local spirits, and illness. These obstacles can make it more difficult to remember dreams as well as create problems in the dream itself.

If you suffer from a problem of prana, the energy in the body is blocked or is in some way prevented from circulating smoothly. Mind and prana are connected; if the prana is disturbed, the mind will be also. In this case, whatever helps you relax before bed, like a massage or hot bath, is an aid. The nine breaths of purification or simply slow, deep breathing can help. Try to remain as calm and relaxed as possible during the day.

The mind can be too busy to allow sleep. For example, after a hectic day it can be hard to stop thinking about it, to let it go; your mind is spread out over problems or excitements and is tight with intensity or anxiety. If you find it difficult to calm the mind, it can be helpful to do hard physical work or exercise to tire the body or even exhaust it. Meditating on emptiness can clear the mind. And, as noted before, taking whatever steps you can to relax before sleep is helpful.

A disturbance with the local spirits can result in broken, restless sleep. I know many Westerners do not believe in such things. They may think the idea of local spirits is symbolic of the energy of a place, the vibe, the feel of the environment. In a way, they are right. But Tibetans believe there really are spirits, beings living in a locale, and if one does something to energetically interfere with those beings, one can be affected by them in return. The provocation of local spirits may result in terrible dreams, the inability to remember dreams, or restlessness that prevents sleep.

For this situation, Tibetans have several remedies. They often go to a shaman and ask for divination to discover the source of the problem and an appropriate action to take. Or they do chöd practice, making offerings to the spirits. They may go to the master and ask for help, which is often given in the form of a ritual that

severs the spirit's connection to them. The master will usually ask
for something belonging to the petitioner, a few hairs or an article of
clothing, and burn it in the ritual fire. Though Tibetans have these
remedies, they are only of benefit if you believe spirits are disturbing you. Otherwise, you won't take the steps necessary to repair
the situation. If you do have the experience of spirits, offer them
compassion. If you do not believe in such things but are sensitive
to the energy of the place, correct it by burning incense and generating compassion. No matter what you believe, the best remedy
is to generate compassion and love for all beings. This will change
the internal environment of your mind and emotions.

The fourth obstacle is illness, and the teaching naturally recommends that you go to a doctor.

No obstacle should discourage you. The same problems have been
encountered and overcome by countless others before you. Rely on
the teachings and your teacher to discover the remedies. They are
available in the teaching. They only need to be applied.

Too Much Seriousness

One obstacle I often see as I teach is too much seriousness. After
all, our practice is to understand everything as a dream. We come
to realize this through the practice of dream yoga. Eventually we
see waking life is also a dream. Then, here you are, being very serious about the dream yoga practice, not seeing the practice as a
dream too. Instead, it seems to be a real obligation or commitment
one has to take seriously. It can cause tension and agitation and
becomes a burden. If you feel like this, your practice is not going to
work.

The whole approach is to relax, take a deep breath, open, allow,
trust. Allow the result of the practice to come to you. Of course, that
doesn't mean you do nothing. Do the foundational practices, the
preparations for night, and the main practices with intent, but also
with openness, ease, a relaxed attitude. If you become frustrated,
you're trying too hard. Allow the result to come to you rather than

working hard to make the result happen. Just let the practice be part of your life.

For example, sometimes I meet people who have a natural ability to have lucid dreams and have some success in the dream yoga practice. When they meet me for the first time, they tell me about lucid dreams they've had, that they saw me in a dream, lots of things. But then they come to a dream yoga workshop and focus for a month, and it all stops. When they see me, I tell them they've gotten too serious about everything. The secret teaching is—relax.

CHAPTER 17

Controlling and Respecting Dreams

Some schools of Western psychology believe it is harmful to control dreams, that dreams are a regulatory function of the unconscious or a form of communication between parts of ourselves that should not be disturbed. This view suggests the unconscious exists and that it is a repository of experience and meaning. The unconscious forms the dream and embeds in it meaning that will be either explicit and obvious or latent and in need of interpretation. In this context, the self is often thought to be composed of the unconscious and conscious aspects of the individual, with the dream being the medium of communication between the two. The conscious self then benefits by working with the dream, mining it for the meaning and insight the unconscious has placed in it. Or the benefit may be from the catharsis of the dream, or from the balancing of physiological processes through the dream-making activity.

Understanding emptiness changes our understanding of the dreaming process. These entities—the unconscious, the meaning, the conscious self—exist as separate things only as useful conceptualizations in our minds.

As mentioned earlier, there are two levels of working with dreams. One involves finding meaning in the dream. This is valued in Tibetan culture and in our practices, agreeing with the many Western psychologies that accord value to dreams. In both the East and the West, it is understood that dreams can be a source of creativity, offer solutions to problems, diagnose ills, and so on. In Tibetan culture, we also look to dreams to connect to guardians and for guidance. But the meaning in dreams is not in the dream images. It is being projected onto the dream by the individual examining the dream and then is "read" from the dream. The process is like making meaning from the images that seem to appear in the ink-spot tests used by some psychologists.

It's easy to think a dream is like a scroll with a secret message written on it in code that, if cracked, anyone could read. But the meaning of the dream will be different from one person to the next and one day to the next; it isn't fixed. There is no conventional meaning outside of an individual mind; meaning does not exist until someone starts to look for it. This view is not giving in to chaos; there is no chaos or meaninglessness either, these are more concepts.

When using dream as an approach to enlightenment, the meaning in the dream is not of primary importance. Although we value insights we receive from dreams, we recognize there is also dreaming in meaning. Dream yoga uses dream to recognize what is below meaning, the pure base of experience. This is the higher dream practice, concerned with recognizing and realizing the fundament of experience, the unconditioned. When you progress to this point, you are unaffected by whether there is a message in the dream or not.

There is no danger of disrupting something important when we change our dreams. All we disrupt is our ignorance.

CHAPTER 18

Simple Practices

Progress in dream and sleep yogas depends on intention, commitment, and patience. There is no single practice to accomplish realization in one night's efforts. Spiritual maturation takes time, and it is in time that we live out our ordinary lives. When we fight time, we lose. But when we know how to be in time, the practice unfolds by itself.

The entirety of dream yoga may seem overwhelming, requiring too much to become a reality in our lives. But it is only this way in the beginning. The practice appears complex because a number of different elements are working in harmony to best support the practitioner, and it is particularly in the beginning of the practice that we need the most support. Take the time to fully understand each element in the preparations and the practices, and use them together to develop experience.

As dream yoga is mastered, the practice becomes simpler and simpler. When awareness is stable, one need not do any of the particular forms of the practice. It's enough to abide in presence and generate intention to cause lucid dreams to arise naturally. Once you are regularly able to be lucid in dream, experiment with simplifying the practice.

For now, even if you choose not to work with the entire practice, there is much that can be done easily, adding simple practices here and there, integrating practice into life gradually until all of life is an opportunity to practice. You needn't abandon the practice if it seems to be too much. Take what you can use from it.

Abiding in clear presence, in awareness, is the essential practice. This practice can be done in any and every moment.

The Waking Mind

We are awake for roughly sixteen hours each day, and the mind is busy the whole time. Often it seems there is not enough time. The world constantly makes demands on our attention—a thousand things can grab our attention and carry it away. The day becomes a blur, leading to weariness and hunger for even greater distraction to escape stress. Living this way is not helpful for any practice, including dream yoga. As an antidote to this scattering, we can cultivate simple and regular habits of reconnecting to ourselves, of becoming more present.

Every breath can be a practice. With the inhalation, imagine drawing in pure, restorative, relaxing energies. With each exhalation, imagine expelling all obstacles, stress, and negative emotions. This is not something that requires a particular place in which to sit. It can be done waiting for a stoplight, sitting in front of the computer, preparing a meal, cleaning the house, or walking. It can change your state in a few minutes.

The mind is like a crazed monkey, ceaselessly jumping from one thought to the next. A simple but powerful practice to develop consistent awareness looks to the body, a source of experience more stable and constant than the conceptual mind. It is always in the present so the attention, when connected to it, stays in the present too.

For example, while walking in a park, the body is in the park, but the mind may be working in the office or at home, talking to a distant friend, planning, or making a list of groceries. The mind has disconnected from the present and the body. Instead, when looking at a flower, really look at it: the color, the shape, the fragrance, the feel. Be fully present. With the help of the flower, the mind returns to the park.

Appreciation of sensory experience reconnects mind and body. It opens the mind to beauty. When experience is unified, a healing occurs, and it is always available. Be present with trees, smell smoke, feel the cloth of your shirt, hear a birdcall, or taste an apple. But also be present with the sound of traffic, the smell of rot, the sight of garbage. Train yourself to experience sensory objects vividly, without judgment. Try to be completely the eye with form, the nose with smell, the ear with sound, and so on. Try to be complete in experience while remaining in just the bare awareness of the sensory object. This will lead to more vivid experience in dreams as well as in waking life.

The practice is simply to try to remain aware of the body throughout the day. If you are not in a situation to focus without interruption, that's okay. Just return awareness to the body frequently during the day. And relax. Feel the body and awareness as a whole. Over time, the mind will grow calmer and more focused.

As the practice of presence is developed, habitual reactions still occur. Upon seeing the flower, judgments about it arise, or a smell may be labeled foul. But there is a moment before an object is given a name, a moment of pure perception. It is always clear and bright. That is pure awareness, your own fundamental nature. Though obscured by the distractions of the mind, it is always there, as the sun is there even when completely covered by clouds.

Being distracted by a cloud of concepts is a habit, and it can be replaced with a new habit. Using the sensory experience of the body to anchor our awareness connects us to the beauty of the world, to the vivid and nourishing experience of life lying under our distractions. Gradually the mind gentles and becomes calmer, and the qualities most conducive to successful dream practice—presence and lucidity—are developed.

Preparing for Night

We may feel half-dead after a stressful day. Later we fall into bed and become almost completely dead. We do not spend even a few minutes to connect body and mind in presence, but spend the evening in distraction, remaining distracted as we prepare for bed and then drift away in sleep. Connecting mind, body, and feeling is one of the most important things we can do to ensure our progression on the spiritual path. We should take a little time to do that each night before sleep.

To have healthier sleep and stronger results in dream practice, spend a few minutes before sleep reconnecting to presence and calm. Simple things are effective: take a bath, burn incense, sit in front of a shrine or in your bed and connect with enlightened beings or your master. Simpler still, and more important, generate feelings of compassion; pay attention to the feeling of your body; cultivate the experiences of joy, happiness, and gratitude. Generating positive thoughts and feelings, fall asleep. The prayers and love will relax the body, calm the mind, and bring contentment and peace to both. Then, feeling secure and at peace, pray: "May I have a clear dream. May I have a lucid dream. May I rest in awareness." Repeat these lines or similar ones you compose with intent, out loud or internally. This is so simple to do, but it will change the quality of your sleep and dreams, and you will be more rested and grounded in the morning.

Make the Practice Simple

If you feel the four stages of practice—the focus on the throat, brow, heart, and secret chakras—are too complicated, just work with the first practice in the throat chakra. Imagine a red, luminous *A* there, after you have prepared for sleep. Focus in the chakra, feel peace, and fall asleep. It is important to have calmed yourself beforehand, to feel connected to the body. If even the concentration on the *A* seems too difficult or complex, then just feel your entire body, relax, connect to presence and compassion. This is the way to clean the mind and the body, which have become stressed and foggy during the day. Every night we brush our teeth and wash if we need to, and we feel better and sleep better. If, instead, we go to sleep feeling unclear and unclean, our sleep and dreams are affected. We all know this about the physical level of our existence but often forget how important it is to feel freshness and connectedness in our minds too. Maybe we should write a sentence on our toothbrushes: "After this, wash your mind."

You can work with breathing as you go to sleep. Try to breathe equally in both nostrils. If the right is blocked, sleep on your left side and vice versa. Gentle the breath and allow it to be smooth and quiet. As suggested earlier, exhale stress and negative emotion; inhale pure healing energy. Do this breath nine times, in meditation posture or while lying down, then focus on the red A in the throat. Feel the A rather than focus on it, merge with it rather than remain separate from it.

Upon waking, if you find you feel better and more rested, feel good about your success. Feel the blessings of the masters and the enlightened beings, the pleasure of your own efforts, and the happiness of following the spiritual path. That happiness will encourage the next night's practice and aid in sustaining and developing the practice continuously.

It is not unusual to find it difficult to relax or to feel compassion or love when going to sleep. If you are in this situation, use your creative imagination. Imagine lying on a beautiful, warm beach or walking in fresh mountain air. Draw up a memory of a person, a child, or a pet you love unconditionally and feel the tenderness and compassion. Let the corners of your mouth lift in just a hint of a smile.

Learn how to fully relax yourself, body and mind, before sleep rather than simply falling down into sleep, driven out of presence by the emotions and stresses of the day. These simple practices can be of great help.

A Simple Lifetime Practice

Dream yoga has been a lifelong practice for many accomplished practitioners. They used the practices taught in this book. But people sometimes want a simpler practice, one that is more universally available. In this case, I recommend the practice of taking inner refuge during the day as an informal practice and before sleep at night as part of both the dream and sleep yogas.

How? All through the day there are challenges that may make you feel agitated, angry, confused, or anxious. Or they can strengthen you. When you encounter one of these challenges, either from outside or in your own mind, take inner refuge through the three doors.

Take refuge in unbounded space by bringing your awareness to the stillness in the body, in which all movement occurs. The second refuge is boundless awareness, which you enter through silence in which all sound arises. The third refuge is authentic warmth; you enter through the spaciousness of mind in which all mind phenomena arise.

There are also three reminders that call you to the practice. They have to do with what I call the pain body, pain speech, and pain mind. What are these?

The pain body is related to the narrowness of your identity with the ego. Your ego is painful in itself, and ego is tied to the body. Anytime someone pushes your buttons, offends you, insults you, or is inconsiderate, it hurts. It hurts the ego, the identity. "You hurt *me*." That "me" is the pain body. When you feel that pain, you react and become impatient or angry, insecure or hurt.

When this discomfort arises, welcome it as a reminder to practice. Immediately connect to your body. Find the stillness inside. Stay present. Allow thoughts and feelings to arise and dissolve. As you practice, remain longer in the stillness and gradually begin to feel more connected to the inner space. You have found your inner refuge. Unbounded space is your protection. It is beyond the anger or anxiety. Rest there. It is the buddha within.

You become aware of the second reminder when you encounter your pain speech. It manifests in your mind when the voice of your thoughts is agitated, irritated, complaining, hurt, anxious—that is pain speech. It is also when your speech causes pain: insulting, belittling, angry, threatening, mocking, or diminishing others. This happens particularly with loved ones. Often we say these things, but we wouldn't if we were fully present, if we weren't driven by conditioning. Practice catching yourself before you say anything. The moment you notice what you're doing, the moment you become aware of the agitation in your head. Don't say it out loud. Let go of the disturbed energy in your head, in your thoughts. Instead, listen to the silence underneath all words, the silence in which all sound arises, the silence within. Your thoughts arise and dissolve in silence. This is a door to inner refuge, to unbound awareness, to the light within. Rest in that awareness. Your pain speech helped you find your inner refuge.

The third door is through the pain mind. Pain mind is what I call the imagination of the distressed ego. The mind is going crazy thinking about something. For example, the mind is thinking about hurting someone or hurting oneself: "I'd like to do this to them/myself!" Thoughts of revenge, of getting even. Rehearsing what you'll say next time or what you wish you'd said last time. Going over and over how you were hurt by someone, how unfair it is, how miserable you are, how terrible they are.

When you're having these thoughts, recognize them as the expression of your pain mind. Let them be a reminder to enter the inner refuge of the mind, the spaciousness in your heart. Immediately draw attention to the heart and feel the spaciousness there. Relax the heart, the chest, and take a deep breath. As you feel spaciousness, the pain mind, no matter how crazy it is, will dissolve. Sometimes this will happen very fast, sometimes it might take a little time. Sometimes it is easy, sometimes more difficult, but give the practice time and the pain mind will eventually dissolve. When it does, rest in the spaciousness of the mind. Become more familiar with it. Eventually you may discover a naturally existing warmth or bliss in the spaciousness of the heart-mind. Abiding in the warmth is the third refuge. So, enter that refuge, reminded by pain mind. The door is the spaciousness in your heart, the refuge is natural warmth. This is the informal practice you should repeat throughout the day.

Very simply, you take painful experience and turn it into practice. Discomfort becomes a guide, directing you to inner refuge, to the clear, luminous awareness that is your fundamental nature. Every time you do this practice, it becomes easier and deeper. You will feel you are nourishing yourself. Ignorance drains us, but awareness nourishes.

Practice as many times as possible during the day. Make it a habit. And practice before sleep. It's very simple. You're in bed. If there is disturbance in your mind or body, use it as a reminder to return to the inner refuge. Draw attention to the stillness in which the body moves, the silence underlying all sounds, the clear spaciousness of the mind in which all experience arises, and the warmth in your heart. If you fall asleep in that, your dreams will be clear.

Taking inner refuge is a lifetime practice. It is not about practicing for three or four weeks. I do it every day.

CHAPTER 19

Integration

Dream practice is not just for personal growth or to generate interesting experiences. It is part of the spiritual path, and its results should affect all aspects of life by changing the practitioner's relationship to the world.

Working with dream practices, we develop presence and positive qualities. We become flexible in life as we become aware of the dreamlike nature of our waking life. Then we can change ordinary life into experiences of compassion and beauty, incorporating everything into the path.

It is when our conventional selves dissolve in clear awareness that we move beyond hope, fear and meaning, beyond the discriminations of positive and negative, beyond trying. Even beyond practice. The nonconventional truth is beyond healing and the need for healing. When we abide in pure awareness, negativities no longer rule us. This makes it easy to test ourselves: how free we are of habitual reactions, how vivid is presence, how undistracted we are, how often we choose kindness as our response to others.

The greater lucidity necessary to progress to this point is naturally brought into the dreams of night. When lucidity is developed and stabilized in dream, it later manifests in the bardo. When one abides in pure awareness in the bardo, liberation is attained.

Apply dream practice without interruption, and the results will manifest in every dimension of life. The result of the full accomplishment of the practice is liberation, but along the way, the practice increases compassion and kindness in us, and life becomes more vivid, full of beauty and delight. If the practice is not changing the quality of your life experience, if you are not more relaxed with less tension and less distraction, if you continue to be easily upset by other people and situations, then investigate the obstacles and apply practice to dissolve them. Consult a teacher if possible. If you experience no progression on the path, then it is best to strengthen your intent. When signs of progress do arise, greet them with joy and let them reinforce your intent. Don't be discouraged if progress is slow. With understanding and practice, it will surely come.

CHAPTER 20

Outlined Synopsis of the Dream Yoga Practices

In this chapter we'll summarize the entire dream yoga practice. For detailed instructions on each step, you can refer to the page references given.

Zhiné (page 77)

If you have time, practice calm abiding (zhiné) during the day. Focus on an object and concentrate. The object can be the breath, a visual object, sounds, or sensations. Even a few minutes of practice, if done regularly and often, strengthens concentration and helps to quiet and focus the mind. This benefits all other practices.

The Four Foundational Practices
Changing the Karmic Traces (page 85)

Try to remain in vivid awareness of the present moment, of all sensory and mental experience. Practice throughout the day or choose to practice strongly for short periods: a minute or two at your desk, the time it takes to walk a block, or while you wash dishes. Determine to visit the practice ten or twenty times each day, as much as you can. Make it a habit.

You will be distracted again and again and again. When you notice, return to awareness, even if only for a few seconds. Try to encounter everything—objects of the senses, people, emotions, your body, mental events—while abiding in vivid, open awareness. Imagine you are in a lucid dream, frequently reminding yourself, "This is a dream." When you do, don't just repeat it: increase the clarity of your awareness and focus on the moment. Is it a dream? Involve your body and senses in becoming more present. Experience will become more vivid and dreamlike as you become lucid in the dream of the day. With consistent practice, you will rest in open awareness more often and for longer periods.

Removing Grasping and Aversion (page 88)

Recognize all you encounter and your reactions to what you encounter as the luminous phenomena of a dream.

Throughout the day, when you notice a negative reaction to people, situations, or your own thoughts, recognize an opportunity to practice. Immediately relax your body and center yourself in clear awareness. Observe the outer situation and what arises in your mind and body. Remind yourself that what you experience is a dream, your reactions are part of the dream, your grasping and aversion are actions in the dream. Recognize this with a level of conviction strong enough to leave an imprint on your mind. Become lucid.

Further the practice by developing flexibility. Let go of habitual responses: stay open, remain aware, and choose to respond positively and with kindness. This will diminish the power of grasping and aversion. You can be certain you are doing this correctly if immediately on seeing your reaction as a dream, desire and attachment lessen.

Strengthening Intention (page 89)

Before going to sleep, review the day and the day's practice. While centered in clear awareness, let memories of the day arise, particularly difficult moments to which you may have reacted. Recognize those events and your reactions as memories of dreams. As in the first two practices, try to truly comprehend and feel the dreamlike nature of your daytime experience.

Develop a strong intention to be aware in the coming night's dreams. Put your heart into this intention. Pray strongly for success or use statements to strengthen your intent: "May I have good sleep. May I have clear dreams and remember them. May I have lucid dreams. May I practice transformation in my dreams."

Cultivating Memory and Joyful Effort (page 91)

In the first moments of waking, review the night. Do you remember your dreams? Were you lucid in dream? Record your dreams in a dream journal while they are fresh in your memory. If you had some success, if you remembered a dream or became lucid in one, allow yourself to experience the joy of it. Always celebrate any success in your practice.

If the practice didn't go well, don't feel discouraged or disappointed; this is part of the path. Instead, begin the day with the strong intention to maintain the practice of the foundations during the day, reinforce the intention to become lucid the next time you sleep if you were not, and to further develop lucidity if you were. Then begin the daytime foundational practices.

Preparation for Night

Nine Purifications Breathing (page 96)

Sitting in meditation posture before lying down to sleep, perform the nine purification breaths.

Guru Yoga (page 100)

Practice guru yoga. Generate strong devotion; pray to the objects of refuge, asking for blessings, guidance, and success in this night's practice. Then merge your mind with the mind of the master, the ultimate master, primordial awareness, your true nature.

Protection (page 104)

Lie down comfortably in the correct posture. Use your imagination to transform the room into a protected, sacred environment. Gentle the breathing, and relax the body. Calm the mind. Let go of stories, fantasies, worries, and plans. Generate a strong intention to have vivid, clear dreams; to remember your dreams; and to recognize the dream as a dream while you are in it.

The Main Practices

Bringing Awareness into the Central Channel (page 109)

Lie on the right side, and gentle the breathing. Connect with clear, open awareness. Relax the body. Particularly relax the throat. Draw attention to the throat chakra. Visualize/imagine/feel four red, luminous lotus petals there. In the center of the petals is the translucent, luminous Tibetan *A* tinged red from the petals. Generate the felt experience of peace. Merge with the peace. Gradually let go of images and imaginings as you allow yourself to fall asleep in peace.

If you wake for any reason during the night, turn your attention to the chakra. Lightly visualize/imagine the petals and the *A*; merge again with peace as you fall back into sleep.

If you become lucid in a dream, practice transforming the dream, your dream body, your identity.

THE INFORMAL PRACTICE. The informal practice is undertaken daily in addition to the foundational practices.

Throughout your day, anytime you have a moment and particularly when you feel anxious, agitated, or emotional, draw clear and open attention to the throat chakra. Relax the throat entirely. Lightly imagine the lotus petals and the *A*. Take a breath, relax the body, calm the mind. Let go. Feel peace spread through your body. It only takes a few moments. Eventually you will become aware of the peace naturally arising as you place your awareness in the throat chakra. Repeat this informal practice throughout the day.

After you have realized results from the first main practice, and when you are ready, move on to the second.

Increasing Clarity (page 111)

After the preparatory practices, lie on your right side in the lion posture as in the first practice. Practice the breathing seven times. Relax the body, and gentle the breath. Draw clear and open awareness to the brow chakra, behind the brow at the point where the eyebrows would meet. Visualize/imagine/feel the tiglé there, white and luminous. Feel it. Be aware of only clarity and luminosity as you merge with it. Allow the white light to dissolve everything. Fall asleep in that experience.

If you wake for any reason during the night, lightly touch on the visualization again, imagine the tiglé, and merge with the luminosity as you fall back to sleep.

If you become lucid in the dream, practice transformation.

THE INFORMAL PRACTICE. Throughout the day, anytime you have a moment and particularly if you feel stuck, blocked, lost, or dull, draw clear, open awareness to the brow chakra inside your head. Lightly visualize/imagine/feel the white tiglé. Imagine the luminosity expanding, filling your head. Feel the naturally arising sense of opening, expansion, increasing luminosity, and vividness of awareness. Repeat the practice many times during the day.

Remember to generate and strengthen your intention in any way you have found effective.

After you have obtained results from the second main practice, and when you are ready, move on to the third.

Strengthening Presence (page 114)

After the preparations for night, lie on your back with a high pillow under the head, upper back, and shoulders. Using a high pillow can help keep sleep light and generate more lucidity in dreams, but being uncomfortable is no help. Avoid an uncomfortable neck position; adjust the position of the pillow and the posture as needed for comfort. Cross the legs loosely. Unlike in meditation posture, the legs can be crossed at the ankle or shin, whatever is most comfortable. It doesn't matter which leg is on top.

Connect with open awareness. Draw attention to the heart chakra, at the level of the heart, in the center of the chest, inside the body. Visualize/imagine/feel there a black, luminous HUNG. It represents the strength of open awareness, the power to remain present without becoming lost. It is the symbol of the unconditioned, nondual awareness. Generate the experience of the stillness and spaciousness of awareness and feel the strength of it, the power to remain present, to not become lost. Focus on the black HUNG in the heart chakra. Breathe deeply, fully, and gently twenty-one times. Merge with the black HUNG and fall asleep

If you wake for any reason during the night, become aware of the heart chakra. Lightly touch on the visualization again; imagine the HUNG; merge with the sense of strength and security, with the stability of clear awareness. Let go into sleep. If you become lucid in your dreams, practice transformation.

THE INFORMAL PRACTICE. When you have a moment, particularly when you feel lost, uncertain, distracted, or tangled up in the stories in your head, draw clear, open awareness to the heart center. Feel the space there. Be open awareness. Feel the strength arise naturally, the stability of being aware of the present. Strengthen your intention to go deeper into the practice in any way you've found effective.

After you have experienced results from the third main practice, and when you are ready, move on to the fourth.

Developing Fearlessness (page 117)

After the preparatory practices, begin the fourth practice. There is no particular posture to take. There is no particular way to breathe except to gentle the breath. Bring open attention to a black tiglé, a luminous sphere of black light, in the secret chakra inside the body. The chakra is behind the genitals, about four finger widths below the navel. The tiglé represents the fearlessness that naturally arises when you rest the mind in open, nondual awareness. Merge with the tiglé. Become awareness. Let go. Gently fall into sleep. When you are lucid in dreams, practice transformations and dissolve boundaries.

Upon each awakening, try to be present and be with the practice. In the morning, immediately be present. Review the night, and record your dreams. Generate intention to continue with the practice during the day.

THE INFORMAL PRACTICE. Throughout the day, when you have a few moments, draw clear, open attention to the secret chakra, especially in moments of anxiety, worry, or fear. Visualize/imagine/feel the black tiglé. If you have experience of it, generate fearlessness and feel the stability of relaxing in open awareness, even if only for a few seconds.

The most important point of the preparations, the foundational practices, and the main practices is to maintain clear awareness, to abide in presence as consistently as possible both day and night. This is the essential practice of both dream and sleep yoga.

PART FOUR

Sleep

The chapters in this section assume the reader has some familiarity with basic tantric terminology. Unlike the earlier material on dream yoga, the teachings on sleep yoga are primarily addressed to those who are already tantric or Dzogchen practitioners and those with strong experience in dream yoga.

CHAPTER 21

Sleep and Falling Asleep

The normal process of sleep occurs as consciousness withdraws from the senses and the mind loses itself in distraction. Mental images and thoughts thin out until the mind dissolves in darkness. Unconsciousness then lasts until dreams arise. When they do, the sense of self is reconstituted through dualistic relationship with the images of the dream until the next period of unconsciousness occurs. Alternating periods of unconsciousness and dream make up a normal night of sleep.

Sleep is dark to us. We are conscious in dreams because the moving mind is active, giving rise to a dream ego with which we identify. In sleep, however, the subjective self does not arise and we do not form memories We are unconscious.

Although we define sleep as unconsciousness, the darkness and experiential blankness are not the essence of sleep. For the pure awareness that is our basis, there is no sleep. If we are able to abide in rigpa rather than the sleep of ignorance, then clarity, peacefulness, and bliss arise. When we develop the ability to abide in that awareness, we find that sleep is luminous. This luminosity is the clear light. It is our true nature.

As explained in previous chapters, dreams arise from karmic traces. Dream yoga develops lucidity in relationship to the dream images, but sleep yoga is imageless. The practice is the direct recognition of awareness by awareness, light illuminating itself. Later, when stability in the clear light is developed, even dream images will not distract the practitioner, and the dream period of sleep will also occur in the clear light. These dreams are then called clear light dreams, which are different than dreams of clarity. In clear light dreams, the clear light is not obscured.

We lose the real sense of the clear light as soon as we conceptualize it or try to imagine it. There is neither subject nor object in the clear light. If there is any identification with a subject, then there is no entry into the clear light. Actually, nothing "enters" the clear light: it is the base recognizing itself. There is neither "you" nor "it." Using dualistic language to describe the nondual necessarily results in a paradox. The only way to know the clear light is to know it directly.

CHAPTER 22

Three Kinds of Sleep

Sleep of Ignorance

Deep sleep is the sleep of ignorance. No matter how many nights we sleep, every night for thirty years or ninety, we cannot finish sleeping. It is necessary for us as samsaric beings; it sustains us. This darkness is "great ignorance" because it is immeasurable.

We experience the sleep of ignorance as a void or blank in which there is no sense of self, no consciousness and no memories are formed. Think of a long, tiring day; rainy weather; a heavy dinner; and the resultant sleep in which there is neither clarity nor sense of self. We disappear. One manifestation of ignorance in the mind is the mental drowsiness that pulls us toward such dissolution in unconsciousness.

Innate ignorance is the primary cause of sleep. The necessary secondary causes and conditions for its manifestation are tied to the body and the body's weariness.

Samsaric Sleep

The second kind of sleep is samsaric sleep, the sleep of dreams. This type of sleep is called "great delusion" because it seems endless.

Samsaric sleep is like going for a walk downtown in a big city, where all manner of things take place: people embrace, fight, chat, and abandon one another; there is hunger and wealth; people run businesses and people steal from businesses; there are beautiful places, ugly places, frightening places. Manifestations of the six realms can be found in any city, and samsaric sleep is the city of dreams, a limitless realm of mental activity generated by the karmic traces of past actions. Unlike the sleep of ignorance, in which the gross moving mind nearly ceases, samsaric sleep requires the active participation of the moving mind.

While the body calls us to the sleep of ignorance, emotional activity is the primary cause of dreams. The secondary causes are actions based in grasping or aversion.

Clear Light Sleep

The third kind of sleep, which is realized through sleep yoga, is clear light sleep. It is also called the "sleep of clarity." It occurs when the body is sleeping but the practitioner is lost in neither darkness nor dreams, but instead abides in pure awareness.

Clear light is defined in most texts as the unity of emptiness and clarity. It is the pure, empty awareness that is the base of the individual. "Clear" refers to emptiness, the mother, the base, kunzhi. "Light" refers to clarity, the son, rigpa, pure innate awareness. Clear light is direct realization of the unity of rigpa and the base, of awareness and emptiness.

Ignorance is compared to a dark room in which you sleep. Awareness is a lamp. No matter how long the room has been dark—an hour or a million years—the moment the lamp of awareness is lit, the entire room becomes luminous. There is a buddha in the flame, the dharmakaya. You are that luminosity. You are the clear light; it is not an object of your experience or a mental state. When the luminous awareness in the darkness is blissful, clear, unmoving, without reference, without judgment, without center or circumference, that is the clear light.

When thought is observed in awareness with neither grasping nor aversion, it dissolves. When thought—the object of awareness—dissolves, the observer or subject also dissolves. In a sense, the object dissolves in the base, and when the subject dissolves, it dissolves in rigpa. This is a risky example in that one may think there are two things, the base and the rigpa; that would be wrong understanding. They are as inseparable as water and wetness. They are described as two aspects of the same thing to aid us in understanding, to relate the teachings to the apparent dichotomy of subject and object. But the truth is that there is never an object separate from a subject; there is only an illusion of separation.

CHAPTER 23

Sleep Practice and Dream Practice

The difference between dream and sleep practice somewhat parallels the difference in the practice of calm abiding (zhiné) when an object is used and when there is no object. Similarly, in tantric practice, dream yoga is used to generate the divine body of the meditational deity (yidam), which is still in the realm of subject and object, whereas sleep yoga develops the mind of the deity, which is clear awareness. In one sense, dream practice is a secondary practice in Dzogchen because it is still working with vision and images; in sleep practice, there is neither subject nor object but only pure awareness, rigpa.

When the student is introduced to Dzogchen practice, practices with attributes are usually taught first. Only after some development of stability is practice without attributes begun. This is because the dominant style of our consciousness has to do with objects of the subject with which one is identified. Because we are constantly identified with the activity of the moving mind, in the beginning our practice must provide something for the mind to grasp. If we are told "Just be empty awareness," the moving mind cannot make sense of it because there is nothing to hold. It tries to make an image of emptiness in order to identify with it, which is not the practice. But if we say that something is to be visualized and then dissolved and so on, the moving mind feels comfortable because there is something for the mind to do. We use the conceptual mind and objects of awareness to lead the mind to awareness without attributes, which is where the practice must go.

For example, we are told to imagine the body dissolving—that sounds fine, it can be pictured. After the dissolution, there is a moment in which there is nothing to grasp. This provides the situation in which the prepared practitioner can recognize rigpa. It is similar to counting down from ten—ten, nine, eight—until zero is reached. There is nothing to grasp in zero, it is the tiglé of empty space, but the movement leads us there. Counting down to emptiness is similar to using practice with attributes to lead us to the emptiness of practice without attributes.

Sleep practice actually has no form, so there is nothing on which to focus. The practice and the goal are the same: to abide in the inseparable unity of clarity and emptiness beyond separation of perceiver and perceived. There are no qualities, no up or down, no inside or outside, no top or bottom, no time or boundaries. There are no distinctions at all. Because there is no object for the mind to grasp as there is in dream, sleep yoga is more difficult than dream yoga. Becoming lucid in a dream means the dream is recognized; it is the object of awareness. But in sleep practice, the recognition is not of an object by a subject but the nondual realization of pure awareness, the clear light, by awareness itself. The sensory consciousness is not functioning, so the mind that relies on sensory experience is not functioning. The clear light is like seeing without an eye, an object, or a seer.

This is analogous to what occurs in death: it is harder to become liberated in the first bardo, the primordially pure (*kadag*) bardo, than in the subsequent bardo, the clear light (*od-sal*) bardo, in which images arise. At the time of death, there is a moment of total dissolution of subjective experience prior to the appearances of the bardo visions. In that moment, there is no subjective self, just as daily experience ends in the dissolution of sleep. We are gone. Then dreams arise in sleep, or images arise in the bardo, and as they are perceived, the force of karmic tendencies creates the sense of a perceiving self experiencing the objects of perception. Caught up again in dualism, we continue in samsaric dream if asleep or continue toward rebirth if in the bardo.

You must decide for yourself which of these practices is most suitable. Dzogchen teachings always stress the importance of knowing yourself, recognizing your capacities and obstacles, and using that knowledge to practice in the manner that will be most beneficial. That said, there are only a few people for whom sleep practice will be easier than dream practice, so I recommend beginning with dream practice. If your mind is still grasping, it makes sense to begin with dream yoga, in which the mind can fasten on the dream itself. After you develop stability in rigpa, sleep practice may be easier to accomplish because there is a strong experience of not grasping, not being a subject, which is the situation in sleep. Another reason I recommend starting with dream yoga is that it can take many years for a practitioner to become lucid in sleep. Practicing for a long time without apparent results may result in discouragement, which can become an obstruction on the path. Once you have some experience in either of the yogas, it is good to continue and reinforce the practice.

The two yogas ultimately lead into one another. When dream practice is fully accomplished, rigpa will manifest in dream. This leads to many dreams of clarity and finally to the dissolution of dreams into the clear light. This is also the fruit of sleep practice. Conversely, when progress is made in sleep yoga, dreams will naturally become lucid, and dreams of clarity will spontaneously arise. Lucid dreams can then be used for developing the flexibility of mind as previously described. Final success in either practice requires that the pure presence of rigpa be recognized and stabilized during the day.

PART FIVE

The Practice of Sleep Yoga

CHAPTER 24

The Dakini Seljé Dö Drelma

The *Mother Tantra* teaches that a dakini is the protector and guardian of sacred sleep. It is helpful to make a connection with her essence, which is also the nature of the practice, so she can guide and bless the transition from unconscious to conscious sleep. Her name is Seljé Dö Drelma (gSal byed gdos bral ma). This translates as "She Who Clarifies Beyond Conception." She is the luminosity hidden inside the darkness of normal sleep.

She is formless in sleep practice itself, but as we are falling asleep, she is visualized as a luminous sphere of light, a tiglé. We visualize light, rather than a form like the syllables used in dream yoga, because we are working on the level of energy, beyond form. We are trying to dissolve all distinctions such as inside and outside, self and other. When visualizing a form, it is the habit of the mind to think of that form as something other than itself, and we must go beyond dualism. The dakini is the representation of the clear light. She is what we already are in our pure state: clear and luminous. We become her in sleep practice.

When we develop a relationship with Seljé Dö Drelma, we connect to our deepest nature. We can further this connection by remembering her as much as possible. During the day we can visualize her in sambhogakaya form: pure white, luminous, beautiful. Her translucent body is made wholly of light. In her right hand, she holds a curved knife, and in her left hand a bowl made from the top of a skull. She abides in the heart center, sitting on a white moon disc that rests on a golden sun disc, which in turn rests on a beautiful blue, four-petaled lotus. As in guru yoga, imagine yourself dissolving into her and she into you, mixing your essence until it is one.

Wherever you are, she is with you, residing in your heart. When you eat, offer her food. When you drink, offer her your beverage. You can talk to her. If you are in a space in which you can listen, let her talk to you. This does not mean you should go crazy, but you can use your imagination. If you have read books on dharma and listened to talks on these topics, imagine her giving you the teachings that you already know. Let her remind you to remain in presence, to cut through ignorance, to act compassionately, to be mindful, to resist distractions. Your teacher or friends may not always be available, but the dakini is. Make her your constant companion and the guide of your practice. You will find that eventually the communication will start to feel real; she will embody your own understanding of the dharma and reflect it back to you. When you remember her presence, the room you are in will seem more luminous, and your mind will become lucid; she is teaching you that the luminosity and lucidity you experience is the clear light that you are. Train yourself so that even feelings of disconnection and the arising of negative emotions automatically remind you of her; then confusion and emotional snares will serve to bring you back to awareness like the bell of a temple that marks the beginning of practice.

If this relationship with the dakini sounds too foreign or fanciful, you may wish to psychologize it. That's fine. You can think of her as a separate being or as a symbol you use to guide your intention and mind. In either case, devotion and consistency are powerful assets on the spiritual journey. You may also do this practice with your yidam, if you do yidam practice, or with any deity or enlightened being; it is your efforts that make a difference in your practice, not the form. But it is also good to recognize that Seljé Dö Drelma is especially associated with this practice in the *Mother Tantra*. There is a long history of practitioners working with her form and energy, and making a connection with the power of the lineage can be a great support.

Imagination is very powerful, strong enough to bind one to the sufferings of samsara for an entire life, and strong enough to make the dialogue with the dakini meaningful. Often practitioners act toward the dharma as if it is rigid, but it is not. The dharma is flexible, and the mind should be flexible with it. It is your responsibility to find how to use the dharma to support your realization. Rather than imagining how the day will go tomorrow, the fight you had with the boss, or the evening ahead with your partner, it may be more helpful to create the presence of this luminous dakini who embodies the highest goal of practice. The important point is to develop the powerful intention needed to accomplish the practice and a strong relationship to your true nature, which the dakini represents. As often as possible, pray to her for the sleep of clear light. Your intention will be strengthened each time you do.

Ultimately, you are to become one with the dakini, which does not mean assuming her form as in tantric practice. It means remaining in the nature of mind, being rigpa in every moment. Remaining in the natural state is both the best preliminary and the best practice.

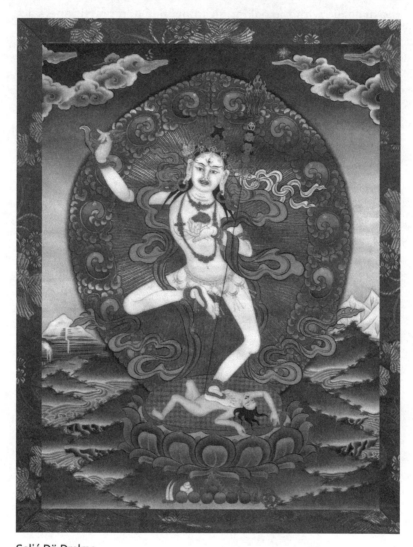

Seljé Dö Drelma

CHAPTER 25

Preliminary Practice

Stress and tension taken to bed will follow you into sleep. Therefore, bring the mind into rigpa if possible. If it is not, then bring the mind into the body, into the central channel, into the heart. The preliminary practices recommended for dream yoga also apply to sleep yoga. Take refuge in the lama, yidam, and dakini, or do the nine breaths of purification and guru yoga. At a minimum, use the mind to promote devotion and practice, such as generating compassion. This, anyone can do. Also pray for clear light sleep. If you have other practices that you normally do before bed, continue doing them.

A small light left on during the night keeps a bit of wakefulness in the mind. It feels different to sleep with a light on, and the difference can be used to help maintain awareness. It's not safe to have a fire of candle burning while you sleep. Battery-powered tea lights, recommended earlier in the book, are good; or a small, dim light.

The light not only helps with maintaining alertness but it also represents the dakini Seljé Dö Drelma. The clarity and luminosity of light are closer to her essence than are any other phenomena in the world of form. When a light is on, imagine the luminosity in the room to be the dakini surrounding you with her essence. Let the external light connect you to the internal light, to the luminosity that is your fundamental nature.

Another preliminary practice is to go without sleep for one or more nights. This exhausts the conventional mind. Traditionally, this is done by a practitioner when the teacher is nearby. After the period of sleeplessness, when the practitioner finally sleeps, the master wakes the practitioner periodically during the night and asks questions: "Were you aware? Did you dream? Did you fall into the sleep of ignorance?"

If you wish to try this, make an arrangement with an experienced practitioner whom you trust. Have the practitioner wake you three times during the night and ask the preceding questions. After each waking, do the practice explained in the next chapter and go back to sleep. Sometimes the conventional mind can become so exhausted that it is very quiet. Then it is easier to find oneself in the clear light.

After your sleepless night it's helpful to receive a massage, if possible, to relax the body and open the channels.

CHAPTER 26

Sleep Practice

Four sessions of sleep practice are scheduled for waking periods in the night, as in dream practice. In sleep yoga, however, all four sessions are the same. If waking four times each night is too disruptive, simply return to the practice whenever you do wake, even if only for a moment, or schedule a single waking at night.

Lie in the lion position on the right side, as explained in the chapters on dream practice. Visualize four blue lotus petals in the heart center. In the center of the petals is the dakini Seljé Dö Drelma, visualized in her essence as a luminous, clear sphere of pure light, a tiglé as transparent as perfect crystal. The tiglé, clear and colorless in itself, reflects the blue of the petals and becomes a radiant whitish blue. Mingle your presence fully with the luminous tiglé to the extent that you become luminous blue light.

On each of the four blue petals is a tiglé, making five with the central one. In front is a yellow tiglé, representing the east. To the left, is the green tiglé of the north. Behind is the red tiglé of the west, and to the right is the blue tiglé of the south. The tiglés represent four dakinis visualized in their luminous essence, the colored light. Do not visualize their forms as anything other than spheres of luminosity. The four tiglés are like a retinue for Seljé Dö Drelma. Develop the sense that you are surrounded by the protection of the dakinis; try to really feel this loving presence until you are secure and relaxed. Pray to the dakinis that you will have the sleep of clear light rather than dreams or the sleep of ignorance. Make your prayer strong and devoted, and pray again and again. Prayer will strengthen devotion and intention. It cannot be overemphasized that strong intention is the foundation of the practice. Developing devotion will aid in making intention one-pointed and powerful enough to pierce the clouds of ignorance that mask the luminosity of the clear light.

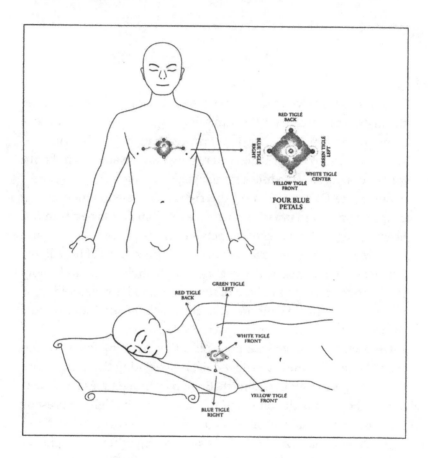

Entering Sleep

Although the experience of falling asleep is continuous, it is divided into five stages as an aid in bringing awareness to the process. In the table below, the column on the left lists a progressive disconnection from the senses and sense objects until there is a total "absence of vision," which here means a complete lack of sensory experience.

Stages in Cessation of Sensory Engagement

Sensory Experience	Tiglé		
	Color	Direction	Location
Vision	Yellow	East	Front
Vision decreasing	Green	North	Left
Vision declining	Red	West	Rear
Vision ceasing	Blue	South	Right
Vision absent	Whitish blue	Center	Center

Normally, identity is dependent on the world of the senses. As that world disappears in sleep, the support for consciousness collapses and the result is "falling asleep," which means we become unconscious. Sleep yoga uses the tiglés to support consciousness as contact with the external world is lost. Corresponding with the progressive dissolution of sensory experience, the practitioner connects to the five tiglés in sequence until, with the external world completely gone, the subject dissolves in the pure luminosity of the clear light. The movement from one tiglé to another should be as smooth as possible in keeping with the continuous and unsegmented movement toward sleep.

Vision. After you lie down in the proper position, sensory experience remains full: you see through your eyes, you hear, you feel the bed, and so on. This is the moment of vision. The conventional self is supported by sensory experience. Begin to shift that support to the pure consciousness that the tiglés represent. The first step is to merge your awareness with the tiglé to the front, a beautiful, warm yellow light in which the conceptual mind can begin to dissolve.

Vision decreasing. When the eyes close, contact with the sensory world begins to diminish. This is the second point, in which vision decreases. As external support is lost, shift awareness to the green tiglé on the left. Allow identity to begin to dissolve as sense experience diminishes.

Vision declining. As sensory experience becomes more muted, shift awareness to the red tiglé to your back. The process of going to sleep is familiar—the softening and blurring of the senses, the gradual loss of sensation. Normally, as the external supports of identity are lost, you lose yourself, but now you are learning to exist without any support.

Vision ceasing. When sensory experience is almost extinguished, move the awareness into the blue tiglé on the right. This is the period when the senses are very quiet and there is barely any contact with the external world.

Vision absent. Finally, as the body completely enters sleep and all contact with the body's senses is lost, awareness fully merges with the central whitish-blue tiglé. By this point, if you are successful, the tiglé will not actually be an object of awareness; you will not visualize a blue light nor will you define experience by location. Rather, you will be the clear light itself; you are to abide in this during sleep.

Notice that these five stages do not refer to inner, mental appearances but to the gradual cessation of sensory experience. Ordinarily, the sleeper moves through this process unconsciously; with this practice, the process is to take place in awareness. The steps in the process should not be clearly demarcated. As consciousness withdraws from the senses, allow the awareness to move smoothly through the tiglés until only nondual awareness—the clear light of the central tiglé—remains. It is as if the body spirals down into sleep while you spiral down into the clear light. Rather than relying on conceptual decisions to move from one tiglé to the next, and rather than trying to make the process happen, allow intention to unfold the process in experience.

If you wake fully in the middle of the practice, start again. You need not be rigid with the form of the practice. Nor does it matter whether the process occurs quickly or slowly. For some people, falling asleep is drawn out; others fall asleep minutes after their head touches the pillow. Both go through the same transition. A needle passes almost instantly through a pile of five gossamer wings, but there are still five moments in which it goes through each in turn. Do not be too analytical about which stage is which or get caught up in dividing the process neatly into five. The visualization is only a support for awareness in the beginning. The essence of the practice is to be understood and applied rather than lost in the details.

In my own experience, I have found the practice is also effective when the tiglés are engaged in the opposite direction. Then, you visualize the yellow tiglé in front, representing earth; the blue tiglé to the right, representing water; the red tiglé to the rear, representing fire; the green tiglé to the left, representing air; and finally the whitish-blue tiglé in the center, representing space. This sequence parallels the sequence in which the elements dissolve in death. You can experiment to determine which sequence works best for you.

As in dream practice, traditionally three more sessions of practice are undertaken during waking periods spaced at roughly two-hour intervals. Once you develop experience, you can use the natural moments of waking in the night rather than scheduled waking periods. Repeat the same practice in each period of waking. Each time you awake, examine the experience of the sleep from which you have just awoken: Did you lack all awareness and thus sleep the sleep of ignorance? Did you dream, lost in samsaric sleep? Or were you in the clear light, abiding in pure awareness?

CHAPTER 27

Tiglé

Tiglé has many different definitions, each appropriate in different contexts. In the context of this practice, it is a small sphere of light representing particular qualities of consciousness or, in the case of the central tiglé, representing rigpa. Although ultimately awareness must be stable without relying on any object, until that capacity is developed, light is a useful support. Light is luminous and clear. Although it is still in the world of form, it is less substantial than any other perceptible object. The visualization of the tiglés is a bridge, a crutch useful until even perceptible light can be abandoned and the practitioner can abide in imageless, luminous awareness.

When you visualize the tiglé on the four blue petals in the heart chakra, it is not necessary to try to determine the exact anatomical site. What is important is to sense the center of the body in the area of the heart. Use awareness and imagination to find the right place, the place in which there is helpful experience.

The colors of the tiglés are not chosen at random. Color affects the quality of consciousness, and the colored lights are meant to evoke particular qualities that are to be integrated in the practice, much as the specific chakras, colors, and syllables form a progression in dream yoga. The different qualities can be experienced as we move from one tiglé to the other—yellow, green, red, blue—to the extent that we allow ourselves to be sensitive to the differences.

This is not a transformation practice in which we would transform our identity; in sleep yoga, identity is given up altogether. It is not the point to stay with a visualization, as it might be in a tantric practice. But the mind must have something to hold; if it does not have the light, it will grab something else.

Before we have experience of rigpa, it is difficult to imagine how we can remain aware with neither a subject nor an object of awareness. Normally consciousness requires an object, which is what is meant by consciousness being "supported" by a form or attribute. Practices in which the visualized object or the subjective identity is dissolved train the practitioner to remain aware as dualistic supports for consciousness disappear. They prepare us for sleep yoga but they are not like sleep yoga itself. Even "practice" is a support. In actual sleep yoga, there is no support and no practice—the yoga is accomplished when the mind that relies on support dissolves into the base.

CHAPTER 28

Progress

Usually when one drives along a familiar route, awareness of the present is lost. Even during a daily commute lasting forty-five minutes or an hour, few things are seen with strong awareness. The driver is on automatic pilot, lost in thoughts, memories, worries, or plans.

Then one becomes a practitioner and decides to remain as present as possible during the drive home, to use the time as an opportunity to strengthen the mind for practice. It is very difficult to do because of conditioning. The mind repeatedly floats away. The practitioner brings it back—to the feel of the steering wheel, the color of the grass along the highway—but this only lasts for a minute before the mind's activity carries the attention away again.

It is the same with meditation practice. The mind is placed on the image of a deity or *A* or the breath; a minute later it wanders off again. It may take a long time, even years, before presence can be maintained continuously for half an hour.

When dream practice is begun, it follows a similar progression. Most dreams are periods of complete distraction; the dream is forgotten almost as quickly as it happens. With practice, moments of lucidity arise, gradually increasing to long minutes of lucid presence in dream. Even then, the lucidity may be lost, or the next dream may again lack lucidity. Progress is made, it is certain and recognizable, but it takes diligence and strong intention.

Sleep practice is usually even slower to develop. But if, after practicing for a long time, there is no progress—no increased presence, no recognizable positive changes in life—it is best not to accept this state of affairs. Rather, one should do purification practices, examine and heal broken commitments (samaya), or work with the prana and energy of the body. Other practices may be needed to clear obstacles and serve as a basis for the accomplishment of dream and sleep yogas.

The practitioner is like a vine that can only grow where there is support. External circumstances have a strong influence on the quality of life, so try to spend time in environments and with people that support your practice rather than detract from it. It helps to read books on the dharma, practice meditation with others, attend teachings, and associate with other practitioners. We have a responsibility to honestly evaluate our practice and its results. If we do not, it is easy to spend many years believing we are making progress when nothing is actually happening.

CHAPTER 29

Obstacles

Sleep yoga is not only a practice for sleep. It is the practice of remaining in clear awareness continually, throughout the four states of waking, sleeping, meditation, and death. The obstacles addressed in this chapter are actually variations of the single obstacle of being driven away from the clear light and into dualistic, samsaric experience. The obstacles are as follows:

1. Losing the presence of the natural clear light of day when distracted by sensory or mental phenomena
2. Losing the presence of the clear light of sleep when distracted by dreams
3. Losing the presence of the clear light of samadhi (during meditation) when distracted by thought
4. Losing the presence of the clear light of death when distracted by the visions of the intermediate state

1. Losing the presence of the natural clear light of day. The obstacle during waking life is external appearance. We become lost in the experiences, the visions, of the sense objects. A sound comes and takes us away; we smell baking and are lost in a daydream of fresh-baked bread; the wind tickles the hair on our neck and we lose the centerless awareness of rigpa and instead become a subject experiencing a sensation as an object. If we remain in the clarity of rigpa, experience is different. A sound arises, but we are connected to the silence in which it arises and do not lose presence.

A vision passes before us but we are rooted in the spaciousness of pure awareness and do not follow the moving mind. The way to overcome the obstacle of external appearance is to develop stability in the natural clear light.

2. *Losing the presence of the clear light of sleep.* The obstacle to realizing the clear light of sleep is dream. When a dream arises, we react to it dualistically and engage in the fiction of being a subject in a world of objects. This is similar to the first obstacle, but it is now internal rather than external. We say images obscure the clear light; however, it is not that the dream actually obscures clarity but that we are distracted from clarity. This is why, in the beginning of practice, we pray to have neither the sleep of ignorance nor the sleep of dream. When we develop enough stability, dream no longer distracts us, and the result is the clear light dream.

3. *Losing the presence of the clear light of samadhi.* The clear light of samadhi is the meditative clear light or consciousness clear light. This is rigpa during meditation practice. Thoughts are the obscuration of the clear light of samadhi. When thoughts arise, we engage them and are distracted from rigpa. The antidote is developing stability in rigpa during practice. Then any thought that arises can be integrated with rigpa; the thought arises and dissolves without distracting us or affecting us.

This should not be taken as an indication that the meditative clear light is only found after many years of practice. In every moment of life, the clear light can be found. Key is whether you are introduced to it and can recognize it with certainty.

4. *Losing the presence of the clear light of death.* The clear light of death is obscured by the bardo visions. The clarity of rigpa is lost when we are distracted by the visions that arise after death and enter into a dualistic relationship with them. As with the other three obstacles, this loss does not have to occur if there is stability in the clear light.

The natural clear light of day is the same as the clear light of night. Knowing the clear light of day, we can find the clear light during sleep. The practice is to connect the natural clear light of waking life to the clear light of sleep and the clear light of samadhi, until we continuously abide in pure rigpa.

The bardo need not obscure the clear light of death. Thoughts need not obscure the samadhi clear light. Dreams need not obscure the clear light of sleep. External objects need not obscure the natural clear light.

If we are deluded by these four obstacles, we will not pass from samsara. Having accomplished sleep and dream practices, we will know how to transform these obscurations into the path. Mystical experiences and insights, as well as all thoughts, feelings, and perceptions, can arise within the presence of rigpa. When they do, allow them to spontaneously self-liberate, dissolving in emptiness, leaving no karmic trace. All experience is then direct, immediate, vivid, and fulfilling.

Sleep practice is not just for sleep; it is the practice of integrating all moments—waking and sleeping, dreaming and in the bardo—with the clear light. When this is accomplished, liberation is the result.

CHAPTER 30

Supportive Practices

This chapter provides short descriptions of practices that support the main sleep practice. Most of them are recommendations from the *Mother Tantra*.

Master

To support the sleep practice and generate stronger devotion to your true nature, imagine the master at the crown of the head and develop connection and devotion. The connection to the master can be based in pure devotion. When you imagine the master, go beyond just visualizing an image: generate strong devotion and feel their presence. Pray with strength and sincerity. Then dissolve the master into light that enters your crown and descends into your heart. Imagine the master abiding there, in your heart center, then go to sleep.

The closeness that you feel to the master is actually the closeness you feel toward your own nature. This is the support of the lama. You may want to reread the section on Guru Yoga found on page 100 for a fuller explanation.

Dakini

On a radiant lotus in the heart, seated on a sun disc that rests on the lotus, abides the dakini Seljé Dö Drelma. She is clear, translucent, and luminous, like a bright light. Feel her presence strongly, feel her compassion and care. She is protecting you, aiding you, leading you. She is the ally that you can wholeheartedly depend upon. She is the essence of the clear light, your goal, enlightenment. Generate love and trust and respect for her. She is the illumination that comes with realization. Focusing on her and praying to her, fall asleep.

Behavior

Go to a quiet place where there are no other people. Cover your body with ashes. Eat heavy foods that help to overcome wind disorders. Then jump around wildly, fully expressing whatever is inside, letting out whatever blocks or distracts you. No one is around, so explode if need be. Let this catharsis clean and relax you. Act out all your tensions. With great fervor, pray to the master, the yidam, the dakini, and the refuge tree; pray strongly, asking for the experience of clear light. Then sleep inside that awakening experience.

Prayer

If you have not had the experiences of the clear light of day, meditation, and sleep, pray for these results again and again. It is easy to forget about the simple power of wish and prayer. We think prayer must be something extraordinary, directed to some incredible power external to us, but this is not the case. The important point is to feel strongly the intent and desire in the prayer, to put your heart in it.

Originally, perhaps, when people wished one another good night or good morning or to sleep well, there was some power in the words, some feeling. Now these are just habitual phrases that we mutter with little feeling or meaning. The same words are used, they are spoken in the same tone, but they are without power. Be careful not to do this with prayer. Know that prayer has power, but it is not in the words; it is in the feeling you put into the prayer. Develop intention, make it strong, and put it into the prayer.

Dissolving

Doing this exercise can give you a sense of how the focusing in the practice should be. The practice begins with light and the perceiver of light, but the intent is to unify the two.

Relax fully. Shut your eyes and begin with a visualization of the whitish-blue tiglé, about the size of a thumbprint, in the heart center. Slowly let it expand and grow more diffuse. It is good to see the light of the tiglé, but it is more important to feel it. Let the light radiate from your heart. As the beautiful blue light shines out, it dissolves everything it touches. Dissolve the room you are in, the house, the town, the state, the country. Dissolve every part of the world, the solar system, the entire universe. Every point the mind touches—whether place, person, thing, thought, image, or feeling—dissolves. The three worlds of desire, form, and the formless dissolve. When everything external is dissolved in light, then let the light come to you. Let it dissolve your body, so the body turns into blue light and merges with the blue light around it. Then dissolve your mind—every thought, every mental event. Dissolve everything. Merge with the light. Become the light. Now there is no inner or outer, no you or not you. There is no sense of a substantial world or self. There is only the luminosity in the space of the heart, which is now pervasive space. Experience still arises; allow whatever arises to dissolve spontaneously in blue light. Let this happen without effort. There is only light. Then slowly dissolve even the light into space.

It is here you should remain during sleep.

Expanding and Contracting

This is a similar but more formal practice meant to support sleep yoga. Visualize thousands of blue HUNGs coming from both nostrils with each exhalation. They originate in the heart and travel up the channels to leave the nostrils with the breath. As they spread out, pervading all space and all dimensions, they dissolve everything they encounter. Their luminosity illuminates all space. With the inhalation, the light of the HUNGs returns, illuminating and dissolving body and mind, until there is no inner or outer. Do this visualization until there is only the expanding and contracting light of the HUNGs. Dissolve into this light and abide in the nondual state. Do this for twenty-one breaths, or more if you like. Practice this during the day as often as possible.

The mind plays tricks. Its main trick is to identify itself as the subject and then take everything else to be separate from that subject. In this practice, everything perceived as outside yourself is dissolved on the exhalation. The perceiver is dissolved on the inhalation. Both outside and inside become luminous and clear and merge into one another, becoming indistinguishable. Whenever the mind finds a path into distraction, let awareness follow after it with blue HUNGs. When the mind reaches for an object, dissolve the object in light. When the mind returns and fixes on itself as a subject, then dissolve that too. Eventually, even the sense of solidity can dissolve, the sense of here and there, of objects and subjects, of things and entities.

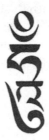

The Tibetan syllable HUNG

Generally we think of doing this kind of practice as an aid in generating clear light experience, but it is also helpful in prolonging the experience once it is known and in supporting the continuity of experience.

CHAPTER 31

Integration

Once we know rigpa, all of life is to be integrated with it. This is the function of practice. Life needs to take some form; if we do not shape it, it will take a form dictated by karma, which we may not like very much. As the practice is increasingly integrated with life, many positive changes will occur.

Integration of Clear Light with the Three Poisons

The clear light must be integrated with the three root poisons: ignorance, desire, and hatred.

Sleep yoga is used to integrate the first, ignorance, with the clear light.

Integrating desire into clear light is similar to discovering the clear light in sleep. When we are lost in the darkness of sleep, the clear light is hidden from us. When we are lost in desire, our true nature is obscured too, but whereas the sleep of ignorance obscures everything completely, even the sense of self, desire obscures rigpa in particular situations. It makes for a strong separation between the subject and the object of desire. The "wanting" itself is a constriction of consciousness arising from the feeling of lack that remains as long as we do not abide in our true nature. Although the purest desire is the longing for the wholeness and completion of full realization, because we do not directly know the nature of mind, desire becomes attached to other things.

If we directly observe desire rather than becoming fixated on the object of desire, the desire dissolves. If we can abide in pure presence, the desire, the desiring subject, and the object of desire will all dissolve into their empty essence, revealing the clear light.

We can also use the satisfaction of desire as a means of practice.

There is joy in the union of emptiness and clarity. In Tibetan iconography, this is represented in the *yab yum* figures, the forms of male and female deities in union. These forms represent the unity of wisdom and method, emptiness and clarity, kunzhi and rigpa. The joy of union is present in any unification of apparent dualities, including the desiring subject and the desired object. At the moment when a desire is entirely satisfied, desire is extinguished. There is a moment in which we are free. When that happens, the clear awareness is exposed, though the force of our karmic habits usually carries us into the next movement of duality, leaving a gap in our experience—almost an unconsciousness—rather than the experience of rigpa.

For example, there is the practice of sexual union. Normally our experience of orgasm is one of pleasant dreaminess, almost unconsciousness, an exhaustion of desire and restlessness that comes about through fulfillment of desire. We can integrate that bliss with awareness. Rather than becoming lost, if we maintain full awareness without separating the experience into an observing subject and the experience being observed, we can use the situation to find the sacred. The moving mind drops away for a moment and reveals the empty base; integrating that moment with awareness, we have the integration of emptiness and bliss that is spoken of particularly in tantric teachings.

There are many such situations in which we normally lose ourselves and can instead be moments in which we find our true nature. We do not become lost only in orgasm or intense pleasure. Even in small pleasures we generally lose presence and become bound in the feelings or objects of pleasure. Instead, we can train ourselves so that pleasure itself is a reminder to rest in full awareness; to bring awareness to the present moment, the body, and the senses; and to let go of distraction. This is one way to integrate desire with clear light, and it is not limited to any particular category of experience; it can be done in any dualistic situation in which there is subject and object. When pleasure is used as a door to practice, the pleasure is not lost; we need not be "anti-pleasure." When the subject and object dissolve in clear light, then the union of emptiness and clarity is experienced and there is joy.

The approach to hatred or aversion is similar. If we observe anger rather than participating in it, identifying with it, or being driven by it, then the obsession with the object of anger ceases and the anger dissolves into emptiness. If presence is maintained in that emptiness, then the subject, too, dissolves. The presence in that empty space is the clear light.

"Observing in pure presence" does not mean that we remain as an angry self, observing the anger, but that we are rigpa, the awareness in which the anger is occurring. When observed in this way, anger dissolves in the empty spaciousness of the mind. That is the clear. But still there is awareness, presence. That is the light. Anger is no longer obscuring the clear light.

Dzogchen is not complicated. The Dzogchen texts often have lines such as, "I am so simple that you cannot understand me. I am so close to you that you cannot see me." When we look far away, we lose awareness of what is close to us. When we look to the future or past, we lose the present.

Tibetans have a saying: "The more wisdom is present, the fewer thoughts there will be." It suggests a two-way process. As practice becomes clear and stable, thoughts will dominate experience less. Some people are afraid of this, afraid that if they let go of anger, for example, they will not address what is wrong in the world, as if they need anger to motivate them. But this need not be true. As practitioners, it is important to be responsible for our conventional lives. When bad things happen, they must be taken care of; when something is wrong, it must be addressed. But if we do not see something wrong, we need not go looking for it. Instead, we remain in the natural state. If we have anger, we must work with it. But if we do not have anger, we are not missing anything of importance.

I meet many people who say they are Dzogchenpas, practitioners of Dzogchen, and are integrated. There is another Tibetan saying: "When I go up to the steep and difficult places in the borderlands, I pray to the Three Jewels. When I come down to the beautiful flowery valley, I sing songs." It is easy to say we are integrated when things are easy. But when a strong emotional crisis comes, it is the test. There is a precision in the practice of Dzogchen. We can discover for ourselves how integrated we are with the practice by paying attention to how we react to the situations that arise in our lives. When a partner leaves, the partner we dearly love, then where do the beautiful words of integration go? We experience pain. Even this must be integrated.

Integration with the Cycles of Time

Traditionally, a practice is discussed in terms of view, meditation, and behavior. This section is about behavior. Behavior is described relative to external, internal, and secret unifications with periods of time.

Generally we lose energy and presence as we move through the day. Instead, in developing the practice, we learn to use the passage of time to move us toward a more stable experience of the clear light.

External Unification:
Integrating the Clear Light into the Cycle of Day and Night

For the purposes of the practice, the twenty-four-hour cycle of day and night is divided into periods that can be used as supports in developing continuity in the clear light of pure presence. People in the past followed schedules set by the natural cycle of day and night, but this is no longer true. If your schedule is different—perhaps, for example, you work at night—then adapt the teachings to your situation. Although the time of day does affect us energetically, we need not believe that the position of the sun determines the experiences described in the teachings. Instead, think about these times of day as metaphors for internal processes. The *Mother Tantra* labels the four periods as follows:

1. Dissolution of phenomena in the base
2. Consciousness reaching nirvana
3. Arising of innate awareness to consciousness
4. Equalizing the two truths during the waking state

1. Dissolution of phenomena in the base. The first period is considered to be the time between sunset and going to bed, the evening. During this period, everything seems to be growing dark. Sensory objects become unclear. The internal sense organs diminish in power. The *Mother Tantra* uses the metaphor of many small rivers moving toward the sea: external phenomena, the senses, the conventional self, thoughts, emotions, and consciousness are moving toward dissolution in sleep, in the base.

You can use imagination to experience this process during the evening. Rather than going toward darkness, move toward the greater light of your true nature. Rather than being fragmented, spread out in the rivers and tributaries of experience and flow toward the wholeness of rigpa. Normally we are connected to the rivers, which are emptying, but the practice is to remain connected to the sea, the base, which is filling. Everything is moving toward the vast, peaceful, radiant sea of the clear light. As night approaches, flow toward completion in nondual awareness rather than toward unconsciousness.

This is the first of the four periods.

2. Consciousness reaching nirvana. The second period begins when you fall asleep and ends when you wake in the morning, traditionally at dawn. Imagine that time—the quietness of it, the stillness. The text says that when everything becomes dark, a light arises. This is similar to a dark retreat, which is very dark when you enter but soon fills with light.

Try to remain in presence during sleep, fully integrated with the clear light. After external appearances, thought, and feeling dissolve into the base, if you remain in presence, it is almost like entering nirvana, in which samsaric experience ceases. It is empty, yet there is bliss. When we realize this, it is the union of bliss and emptiness. This is seeing the light in the darkness.

It is not that you should wait until sleep to have clear light experience. Try to abide in the clear light before falling asleep. Even while working with the visualizations of sleep yoga, remain in rigpa, if possible.

This is the second period, in which the senses and consciousness are like a mandala of the clear sky. Contemplate in that state as much as possible until morning.

3. *Arising of innate awareness to consciousness.* The third period starts when you wake from sleep and continues until the mind is fully active. The text says that this period lasts from dawn until the sun comes out. Imagine the quality of that time: the first glimmers of light appear in the dark sky and expand into the beauty of the day. The quiet fills with the sounds of activity, of birds or traffic or people. Internally, it is the movement from the quiet of sleep to full engagement with daily life.

The teachings recommend arising very early in the morning. Wake, if possible, in the nature of mind rather than in the conventional mind. Observe without identifying with the observer. This can be a little easier in the first moments of waking because the conceptual mind is not totally awake yet. Develop the intention to wake in pure presence.

4. *Equalizing the two truths during the waking state.* The fourth period begins when you are fully engaged with the day and ends with sunset. This is day, the time of activity, being busy, and relating to other people. It is full immersion in the world, in forms, language, feelings, smells, and so on. The senses are completely active and occupied with their objects. Still, you should try to continue in the pure presence of rigpa.

Losing yourself in experience, you are confounded by the world. But abiding in the nature of mind, you will find no question to be asked or answered. Abiding in nondual presence satisfies all questions. Knowing this one thing cuts all doubt.

This is the fourth period, in which conventional and ultimate truth are equalized in the unity of clarity and emptiness.

Internal Unification:
Integrating the Clear Light into the Sleep Cycle

The progression described here is similar to that in the previous section. Rather than addressing the twenty-four-hour cycle, it focuses on developing continuity of presence during a single cycle of waking and sleeping, whether it is a nap or an entire night. Before going to sleep, we must remember that we have the opportunity to practice. This is something positive, something we can do for both practice and health. If the practice feels like a burden, it is better not to do it until we develop inspiration and joyful effort.

Again, there are four periods:

1. Before falling asleep
2. After falling asleep
3. After waking and before becoming fully engaged in the activities of the world
4. The period of activity until the next period of sleep

1. Before falling asleep. This spans the time from the moment of lying down until sleep comes. All experience is dissolving into the base; the rivers flow into the sea.

2. After falling asleep. The *Mother Tantra* compares this to the dharmakaya, the clear light. The external world of the senses is void, yet awareness remains.

3. After waking. The clarity is there, the grasping mind is not yet awake. This is like the perfected sambhogakaya, void but with total clarity.

4. The period of activity. When the grasping mind becomes active, that very moment is similar to the manifestation of the nirmana-kaya. Activities, thoughts, and the conventional world "start," yet clear light is retained. The world of experience manifests in our awareness.

Secret Unification: Integrating the Clear Light with the Bardo

This practice has to do with integrating the clear light with the intermediate state after death, the bardo. The process of death parallels the process of falling asleep. It is here divided into four stages similar to those of the preceding sections.

1. Dissolution
2. Arising
3. Experiencing
4. Integrating

1. Dissolution. In the first stage of death, as the elements of the body begin to disintegrate, sensory experience dissolves, the energies of the internal elements are released, the emotions cease, the life force dissolves, and consciousness dissolves.

2. Arising. This is the first bardo after death, the primordially pure (kadag) bardo. This is like the moment of falling asleep, ordinarily a period of unconsciousness. The accomplished yogi can release all identities and become liberated directly into the clear light at this stage.

3. Experiencing. The bardo of visionary experience arises, the clear light (od-sal) bardo. This is similar to arising from the blankness of sleep into a dream, when consciousness is manifest in various forms. Most people will identify with one part of the experience, constituting a self, and react to the apparent objects of consciousness, just as in a samsaric dream. In this bardo, too, the prepared and accomplished yogi can attain liberation.

4. Integrating. Next is the bardo of existence, *sidpa* bardo. The prepared practitioner unifies conventional reality with rigpa. This is again the equalization of the two truths, conventional and absolute. If this capacity has not been developed, the individual identifies with the delusory conventional self and relates dualistically to the projections of mind that make up the visionary experience. Rebirth in one of the six realms is the result.

These four periods are stages in the process of dying. We must be aware within them to connect to the clear light. When approaching death, we should, if possible, abide in rigpa before sensory experience begins to dissolve. Do not wait until entering the bardo. When vision has gone but hearing remains, for example, it is a signal to be completely present rather than to be distracted by the other senses. Completely let go into rigpa; this is the best preparation for what is to come.

All the dream and sleep practices are, on one level, preparations for death. Death is a crossroads: everyone who dies goes one way or another. What happens depends on the stability of the practice. Even in a sudden death, such as in a car crash, there is a moment in which to recognize that death has come, even though it may be harder to do so. Right after that recognition, one must try to integrate with the nature of mind.

Many people have had near-death experiences. They say that afterward the fear of death is gone. This is because they have lived that moment, they know it. When we think about the moment of death, we are not living the reality but are in a fantasy of it that contains more fear than does the actual moment. When the fear goes, integrating with the practice becomes easier.

The Three Unifications: Conclusion

All three of these situations—the cycle of the twenty-four-hour day, the cycle of sleeping and waking, and the process of death—follow a similar sequence. First there is dissolution; then the dharmakaya, emptiness; then the sambhogakaya, clarity; then the nirmanakaya, manifestation. The principle is always to remain in nondual presence. The division of processes—as in the dream and sleep yogas—is simply to make it easier to bring our awareness into the passing moments, to give us something to look toward, to train us to use inevitable experiences as a support for the practice.

There is no break in the natural state of mind unless we break from it. To connect all experience to the practice, be aware. Of course, secondary circumstances can be helpful for practice; that is why time is introduced as a secondary circumstance. The early morning is helpful, or the day after not sleeping, or when we are exhausted, or when we are completely at rest. There are many moments conducive to integration, such as the moment of release we feel when we really need to go to the toilet and go, or when a difficult job finally ends, or when we are completely exhausted from carrying something heavy and then put it down and rest. Even every exhalation of breath, if it is done with awareness, is a support for the experience of rigpa. We have to bring ourselves to that which is always awake; then we can wake up what is dreaming and sleeping. When we are identified with what grows tired and falls asleep, wakefulness is obscured. But clouds never truly obscure the light of the sun, only the one who is perceiving the sun.

CHAPTER 32

Continuity

Because we habitually identify with the fabrications of the mind, we do not find the clear light during sleep. For the same reason, our waking life is distracted, dreamy, and unclear. Rather than experiencing pristine awareness, we remain trapped in the experiences of fantasy and mental projections.

Yet awareness is continuous. Even when asleep, if someone softly says our name, we hear and respond. During the day, even when we are most distracted, we remain aware of our environment; we do not walk into walls. In this sense, there is always presence; but the awareness, though unceasing, is foggy and obscured. Piercing the obscurations of ignorance at night, we enter and abide in the radiant clear light. And if we pierce the delusions and hazy fantasies of the moving mind during waking life, we find the same underlying pure awareness, our buddha-nature.

The only limits to practice are those we create. It is best not to compartmentalize practice into periods of meditating, dreaming, sleeping, and so on. Ultimately, we practice to abide in rigpa in all moments, waking and sleeping. Until then, the practice should be applied in every moment. It is not that we must do every practice we learn. Experiment with the practices, try to understand their essence and methods, then discover which practices actually further development and do those until stability in rigpa is attained. The components of the practice are provisional. The position of the body, the preparations, the visualizations, even sleep itself, are not important once one directly knows and abides in the clear light.

The experience of clear light is reached through the particulars of the practice, but once it is reached, there is no need for practice. There is only clear light.

PART SIX

Elaborations

What follows is additional commentary relevant to dream and sleep yoga.

CHAPTER 33

Context

The connection between student and teacher is of central importance in Dzogchen. The student receives teachings, instruction, and transmission from the teacher. As the practice of dream and sleep yoga progresses, understanding the central points of the teachings helps the practitioner stay directed. The nature of the mind cannot be captured in concepts, but without some understanding of the teachings it is difficult to recognize what must be recognized. With a clear understanding, the practitioner can check their experience against the teachings and develop certainty. If possible, these experiences should be checked against the oral teachings given by a teacher during the course of an ongoing relationship.

Though helpful, conceptual understanding is not enough. Without experience, the teachings are abstract philosophy or dogma. It would be like learning about medicine but not treating one's own illness. Knowing the view is recognizing the nature of mind experientially: the practitioner learns what rigpa is by being rigpa. Abiding in the view is not thinking about the teachings but resting in the nature of mind. One discovers the wisdom beyond the conceptual mind by discovering that one's fundamental nature is that wisdom.

CHAPTER 34

Mind and Rigpa

Liberation from ignorance and suffering occurs when we recognize and abide in our true nature. Our necessary task is to distinguish, experientially, the conceptual mind from the pure awareness of the nature of mind. Practice and instruction are needed because, as is written in Dzogchen texts: "I am so simple you cannot understand me. I am so close to you that you cannot see me."

Moving Mind

The conceptual or moving mind is the mind of everyday experience, constantly busy with thoughts, memories, images, fantasies and internal narratives. It is what we normally think of as "me" and "my experience." Our sense of identity is created and maintained in the activity of the moving mind as we take ourselves to be a subject in a world of objects. The moving mind is reactive, wildly so sometimes, but even when calm and subtle—for example, during meditation or intense concentration—it maintains the internal posture of an entity observing and separate from its environment. Its essential characteristic is to instinctively divide experience into subject and object, self and not self.

The *Mother Tantra* refers to this mind as the "active manifestation mind." If the moving mind becomes completely still, it dissolves into the nature of mind and does not arise again until activity reconstitutes it.

The conceptual mind is not an obstruction in itself. Without it we would not be able to function; we would not be fully human. The problem is not the conceptual mind but our identification with it and our ignorance of and distraction from the nature of mind. This misidentification is what the ego is. Through it, we live in internal narratives, cut off from direct experience of the radiance of life that is available to us at any moment we let go of the moving mind and rest in the clear awareness from which it arises.

Rigpa

Rigpa means "awareness" or "knowing." In Dzogchen the word has additional significance as it refers to the fundamental nature of the mind; the primordially pure awareness underlying all experience, and to the recognition of that nature. It is empty of identity yet cognizant, luminous. Its activity is ceaseless manifestation: phenomena endlessly arise without disturbing it. It is this awareness we realize through practice. Unrecognized, the nature of mind manifests as the moving mind. When it is known directly, it is both the path to liberation and liberation itself.

Phenomena arise in awareness like the empty reflections arising in a mirror. Thoughts, images, emotions, sense perceptions—everything. Without light, there is no appearance in a mirror; without awareness, there is no experience. The moving mind itself is an empty appearance in awareness. Identifying with the moving mind, we live as one of the reflections in the mirror, reacting to empty appearances, suffering confusion and pain. We take the reflections for the reality and spend our lives chasing illusions. When the mind is free of grasping, aversion, dullness, and distraction, it relaxes into unfabricated awareness. When there is no identification with the empty appearance of the conventional self, we effortlessly accommodate all that arises. We are not distracted by phenomena in the world or mental phenomena: they do not distract us and we can respond rather than react. All states and all phenomena—even anger, jealousy, and so on—dissolve in the purity and clarity from which they arose. If hatred arises, the mirror fills with hatred. When love arises, the mirror fills with love. For the mirror, love and hate are equally manifestations of the mirror's innate capacity to reflect.

Stabilizing in rigpa makes it easier to realize all other spiritual aspirations. It is easier to practice virtue when free of grasping and the sense of lack, easier to feel compassion when not obsessed with ourselves, easier to practice transformation when free of constricted identities.

The result of abiding wholly in the nature of mind is the three bodies (*kayas*) of the buddha: the dharmakaya, which is the unbounded spaciousness of the primordial, nondual mind; the sambhogakaya, which is ceaseless manifestation of dreamlike phenomena; and the nirmanakaya, which manifests as spontaneous, undeluded compassionate activity.

Abiding in rigpa, we cut karma at its root. This is the mirror-like wisdom.

Base Rigpa and Path Rigpa

In the context of practice we talk about base rigpa and path rigpa. The base rigpa is the pervasive foundational awareness of the kun-zhi (*khyabrig*). All beings with mind have this awareness, buddhas as well as samsaric beings. Buddhas abide in this awareness but it is obscured in unenlightened beings.

Because our minds arise from this primordial awareness, it is our own nature and we can know it directly. When we do, it is called the arising innate awareness of the path (*sam-rig*). This is the individual's experience of the innate awareness. It is called path rigpa because it refers to the direct realization of rigpa that yogis have when they enter the practice of Dzogchen or Mahamudra and receive the introduction.

The primordial base rigpa is always present: it is presence. But our experience of it on the path is intermittent until we are fully liberated. The first is like cream and the second like butter: they are the same, but something must be done to produce the butter.

This is arising or path rigpa because we recognize it in practice then, distracted, reidentify with the moving mind. Our experience is intermittent.

CHAPTER 35

The Base: Kunzhi

The kunzhi is the inseparable unity of emptiness and clarity, of the absolute open indeterminacy of ultimate reality and the unceasing display of appearance and awareness. The kunzhi is the basis or ground of being. It is the limitless space of unbound awareness in which all phenomena arise as empty appearances. Kunzhi has neither inside nor outside; it cannot be said to exist (for it is nothing) or not to exist (for it is being itself). It cannot be destroyed or created, was not born, does not die.

The kunzhi is empty like the sky, but unlike the sky, it is cognizant. This is the clarity or luminous aspect of the kunzhi: awareness. This is not to suggest that kunzhi is a subject "aware of" objects as separate entities. Rather the kunzhi is the unbound awareness in which all things arise as essenceless, dreamlike appearances. The emptiness is the clarity, the clarity is the emptiness.

When the sun goes down in the evening, we say darkness falls. This is darkness from the perceiver's point of view. Space is always clear and pervasive; it does not change when the sun rises or sets; there is not dark space and light space. It is only dark or light for the perceiver. When the lamp of awareness is lit in the practitioner, the space of kunzhi is illuminated, but the kunzhi was never dark. The darkness was our awareness entangled in the ignorant mind.

(The kunzhi in the Dzogchen teaching is not synonymous with the kunzhi as it is referred to in the sutric Cittamatra school, where kunzhi (*alayavijnana*) describes a neutral but unawakened mental consciousness containing all categories of mental activity and karmic traces.)

Mind and Matter

Kunzhi underlies all, so why can sentient beings become enlightened and matter cannot? In Dzogchen we explain this with a crystal and a lump of coal.

When the sun shines, the coal, even when drenched in light, does not become luminous. It lacks the capacity. But when sunlight reaches a crystal, the crystal fills with light and reflects it in multi-hued displays. Crystal has the capacity to reflect; that is its nature. Similarly, while matter lacks the reflective capacity of innate awareness, the fundamental nature of sentient beings is innate awareness. The minds of sentient beings reflect the light of primordial awareness, and its potential is displayed in either the projections of mind or the pure light of rigpa.

CHAPTER 36

Knowing

Much of sutric Buddhism teaches that the ordinary person cannot know emptiness through direct perception but must rely on inferential cognition. In most sutric traditions there is discussion regarding how to employ inferential cognition and reason toward the recognition of emptiness but little about recognition of the nature of mind through the senses. In sutra, only the yogi who has attained the third path, the path of seeing, has yogic direct perception of emptiness, at which time that yogi is no longer categorized as an ordinary being.

Dzogchen teachings tell us that not only can the nature of mind be directly apprehended in sensory experience but that it is easier and more valid to use the senses in this task than to use the intellect. The senses are the immediate gates of direct perception, which, before it is interpreted by the conceptual mind, is very close to pure awareness.

The conceptual mind does not directly experience the world. Instead, it creates models and projects them into experience, mistaking them for reality. For example, we see a table when light is reflected from the table, enters the eye, is processed in the brain and experience arises in the mind as an image. We think we are seeing a table that exists outside of us but what we are experiencing is a mental image of a table. When the eyes are closed, the table can no longer be directly perceived and that set of phenomena is no longer part of the experience of the immediate sensory present. But the conceptual mind can still project an image of the table. It does not need to stay oriented in the physical present but can interact with its own fabrications, as we experience every night in dream and every day in the stories we tell ourselves and in memories.

Even with raw perception, we are normally identified with a perceiving subject and the experience remains dualistic. But in the very first moment of contact between awareness and the object of the senses, the naked nature of mind is there. For instance, when we are sharply surprised there is a moment when all our senses are open: we have not identified ourselves as the experiencer or the experience, no story is being told in the mind. Normally the moment is a kind of unconsciousness because the moving mind with which we identify has, just for that moment, been shocked into stillness. Often people say they "went blank." In that moment, there is neither perceiver nor perceived, only pure experience: no thought, no mental process, no reaction on the part of a subject to the stimulus of an object. There is only open awareness. That is the fundamental nature of mind. To recognize and rest in it is rigpa.

CHAPTER 37

Recognizing Clarity and Emptiness

Recognizing rigpa is not having some kind of peak experience. It is not something found by performing an action or by altering oneself. It is not a trance or visions of light. It is direct recognition of what we already have, what we already are. When there is expectation about rigpa, it cannot be found. The expectation is a fantasy; we look past what is present.

There is little we can say about space, so we normally describe it in terms of what is in it or what it isn't. This is similar to the way we talk about empty clarity, awareness. Though it is the foundation of all phenomena, nothing can be affirmed about it because it has no qualities, attributes, or references. Rigpa cannot be worked with. It is found when the mind is relaxed and no effort is made. When thoughts are let go, when the moving mind is let go, when the self is let go; there is rigpa. If we do not know rigpa where we are right now, we cannot find it until we stop looking for it. It is here, closer to us than our thoughts. It is the ground of experience.

So when we refer to the "experience of clear light," what is meant? It is not an experience we create through practice. The practice is recognizing the unbound, centerless awareness in which all experience arises and into which it dissolves. When the moving mind dissolves in pure awareness, we realize what we already are. This is the son rigpa knowing the mother rigpa; awareness knowing itself.

Discrimination

As practitioners we ask ourselves whether we know rigpa directly in the moment or are distracted from it by the moving mind. No one else can tell us the answer.

The *Mother Tantra* refers to the nature of mind as "primordial mind." It is likened to the ocean, whereas ordinary mind is like a series of waves, temporarily identifiable as this wave or that wave though never being anything other than the ocean. The moving mind is also compared to bubbles in the ocean of primordial mind, forming and dissolving depending on the strength of the karmic winds while the nature of the ocean does not change.

Though rigpa can't be captured in words, the teachings suggest the practitioner check their experience of rigpa against these qualities. Rigpa is like the early morning sky: vivid, pristine, expansive, clear, fresh, quiet, empty. Rigpa is like space: empty, unmoving, unstained, unlimited, unaffected by what arises in it.

CHAPTER 38

Self

The word *self* has been defined differently by various religions, philosophies, and sciences from ancient times to the present. Bön-Buddhism places emphasis on the doctrine of no-self or emptiness (*sunyata*). Without understanding emptiness, it is difficult to cut the root of the egoic self and to find liberation from its boundaries.

But when we read about the spiritual journey, we also read about self-liberation and self-realization. And we certainly seem to be selves. We can argue that we do not have selves, but when our lives are threatened or something is taken from us, the self we claim does not exist can become quite afraid or upset.

According to Bön-Buddhism, the conventional self exists. Otherwise no one would create karma, suffer, and find liberation. It is the inherent self that does not exist. Lack of an inherent self means there is no core discrete entity that is unchanging through time. Though the nature of mind does not change, it is not a discrete entity, a "self." The nature of mind is not an individual's possession and is not an individual. It is the nature of sentience itself and is the same for all sentient beings.

Again, there is the example of reflections in a mirror. If we focus on the reflections, we can say there is this reflection and that other reflection, pointing to two different images. They grow larger and smaller, come and go, and we can watch them embrace each other, show emotion and work at a desk as if they were separate beings. They are like the conventional self; the reflections are not discrete entities; they are a play of light in the empty luminosity of the mirror.

They exist as separate entities only through conceptualizing them as such. The reflections are a manifestation of the nature of the mirror, just as the conventional self is a manifestation that arises from, abides in, and dissolves back into the empty base of pure awareness.

Imagine filling out forms with information about yourself. You list your name, gender, age, address, job, and relationship status. You take tests that describe your personality traits and write down your goals and dreams, beliefs, thoughts, values, and fears. Now imagine all that is taken away. What is left? Take away more—your friends and home, your country and clothes. You lose the ability to speak or to think with language. You lose your memories. You lose your senses. Where is your self? Is it your body? What if you lose your arms and legs, live with a mechanical heart and a lung machine, suffer brain damage and lose mental functions. At what point do you stop being a self? If you keep peeling away layers of identity and attributes, at some point there is nothing left.

You are not the self you were as a young child. There is nothing that does not change. At death, the last remnants of what seems to be an unchanging self are gone. When reborn, you may be a different type of being altogether, with a different body, different gender, different mental capacity. It is not that you are not an individual—obviously you are—but that all individuals lack independent existence. The conventional self exists as a moment-to-moment fabrication, like the reflection in a mirror or the stream of thoughts that endlessly arise in the mind. Thoughts exist as thoughts, but when they are examined in meditation, they dissolve into the emptiness from which they arose. It is the same with the conventional self: when deeply examined, it proves only to be a conceptual construct ascribed to a constellation of constantly changing events. Just as thoughts continue to arise, so do our provisional identities. Erroneously identifying with the conventional self and taking oneself to be a subject in a world of objects is the foundation of dualistic vision and the root of samsara.

When we abide in our true nature, the dream that is our conventional self dissolves into emptiness and luminous clarity. And we wake.

Final Words

The yogas of dream and sleep are not common practices for Tibetans. They have not traditionally been given to young practitioners or taught widely. But things have changed. I am teaching these practices because so many people in the West have an interest in dreams, dreaming, and dream work. Usually this interest is psychological. I hope that by presenting these teachings, dream work may progress to something deeper. Psychological dream work can create more happiness and satisfaction in samsara and that is good, but if full realization is the goal, there is something more. This is where sleep yoga is particularly important. It is at the heart of the practice of the Great Perfection, Dzogchen, which could be summarized thus: every moment of life—waking, dreaming, and sleeping—abide in pure awareness. This is the certain road to enlightenment and the path that all realized masters have taken. This is the essence of sleep yoga.

How can you have the experience of clear light? I think it is important to reflect on this question as it has to do with your attitude toward the teaching. All the teachings are of a single essence. I am referring to rigpa, to the clear light. No matter how much you learn, how many texts you study, how many teachings you receive, you will not have gotten the main point if you do not directly know the fundamental nature of your own mind. Tibetans have a saying: "You can receive so many teachings that your head is flat from being touched with the initiation vase, but if you don't know the essence, nothing will change."

When one does not directly have this recognition, the teachings may seem to refer to something impossible because the nature of mind is beyond the conceptual mind and cannot be comprehended by it. Trying to grasp the nature of mind through concepts is like trying to understand the nature of the sun by studying shadows—something can be learned, but the essence remains unknown. This is why practice is necessary, to go beyond the moving mind and to know the nature of mind directly. It is available in every moment.

Some people come to feel burdened by all the teachings they accumulate. This is based on a misunderstanding of the path. Continue learning and receiving teachings, but develop a deep enough understanding that you can take from them what supports you. The teachings are not an obligation once you understand and apply them. They are a path to freedom, and there is joy in following that path. They may feel like a burden if one becomes mired in their forms without realizing their purpose experientially.

Do not allow yourself to become trapped by the practice. What does this mean? If you continue to practice for a long time without results, with no positive changes, the practice is not effective. Simply going through the motions without understanding, experience, and benefit accomplishes little. You need to penetrate the practice with understanding, determine what the essence is and how to apply it.

The dharma is flexible. This does not mean that you should throw out the tradition. The practices are powerful and effective. They have been the vehicle for countless people to realize liberation. If there are no results from the practice, experimentation should be undertaken to try to find the purpose of the practice and how to progress. Consulting with your teacher is best. When you understand the practices, you will see that the form is not the problem; it is the application of the form that needs to be perfected.

The practice is here for you, not you for it. Learn the form, understand the purpose, apply it in practice, and realize the result.

Where do you ultimately conclude the practice? In the process of death, the intermediate state, the bardo. The bardo after death is like a major airport that everyone has to pass through on their travels. It is a borderline between samsara and nirvana. The capacity to abide in nondual presence is the passport that allows entry to nirvana. If you can integrate with the clear light of sleep, then you can integrate with the clear light of death. Integrating with the clear light of death means finding buddha within yourself and being able to realize directly that what arises is essenceless appearance.

The presence of rigpa continues from this world into the next, so practice to experience it now, to become it and abide in it. That is the path; the continuity of clarity and unceasing wisdom. All the beings who achieved enlightenment and became buddhas crossed the border and entered the clear light. Know this so that you know what it is you are preparing for. Try to get the sense of the whole of the teachings, where you are, and where you are going. Then you will know how to practice correctly and what the results will be. The teachings are like a map that can tell you where to go, where to find what you are looking for. The map clarifies everything. Without it, you can become lost.

Great masters have written that they practiced steadily for many years to accomplish sleep yoga, so do not be discouraged if you have no experience the first or the hundredth or the thousandth time you try it. There are benefits just from doing the practice. Continuity is the key and with awareness and intention, continuity can be developed.

The clear light is the highest joy and the greatest peace. Every individual experiences at least some moments of peace and joy, so, if the clear light seems a distant goal, just try continuously to maintain the experience of peace and joy. Perhaps when you remember the master or the dakini, you feel joy, or when you attend to the beauty of the natural world you feel peace. Make doing these things a practice. Then practice generating joy and peace in increasing difficult situations and moods, and as often as possible. Feel these qualities in the body, see them in the world and wish them for others. Maintain this practice consistently and you will develop flexibility of mind just as you do in lucid dreams: by intentionally changing experience and identity. As you progress, you will be happier and become a positive influence on the life around you. Most importantly, use this practice to develop stability continuity in clear awareness. This is the essential practice.

Bring your entire being to the practice; with strong intention and joyful effort, you will surely find your life changing in positive ways and will certainly accomplish the practices.

I hope that those who have read this book will discover a new knowledge of dream and sleep, one that will help improve their daily lives and ultimately lead to liberation.

Glossary

bardo (Tib., *bar do*; Skt., *antarabhāva*). *Bardo* means "in-between state" and refers to any transitional state of existence—life, meditation, dream, death—but most commonly to the intermediate state between death and rebirth.

Bön (Tib., *bon*). Bön is the indigenous spiritual tradition of Tibet that predates Indian Buddhism. Although scholars disagree about its origin, the tradition itself claims an unbroken lineage that is seventeen thousand years old. Similar to Tibetan Buddhist sects, particularly the Nyingma, Bön is distinguished by a distinctive iconography, a rich shamanistic tradition, and a separate lineage reaching back to Buddha Shenrab Miwoche rather than to Shakyamuni Buddha.

The nine vehicles of Bön contain teachings on practical matters, such as grammar, astrology, medicine, prognostication, the pacification of spirits, and so on, as well as teachings on logic, epistemology, metaphysics, the different levels of tantra, and complete lineages of the Great Perfection (Dzogchen).

chakra (Tib., *khor-lo*; Skt., *cakra*). Literally, "wheel" or "circle." *Chakra* is a Sanskrit word referring to energetic centers in the body. A chakra is a location at which a number of energetic channels (tsa) meet. Different meditation systems work with different chakras.

channel (Tib., *tsa*; Skt., *nādi*). The channels are the "veins" in the system of energetic circulation in the body, through which stream the currents of subtle energy that sustain and vivify life. The channels themselves are energetic and cannot be found in the physical dimension. However, through practice or natural sensitivity, individuals can become experientially aware of the channels.

chöd (Tib., *gcod*). Literally, "to cut off" or "to cut through." Also known as the "expedient use of fear" and the "cultivation of generosity," chöd is a ritual practice meant to remove all attachment to one's own body and ego by compassionately offering all that one is to other beings. To this end, the practice involves an elaborate evocation of various classes of beings and the subsequent imaginary cutting up and transformation of the practitioner's body into objects and substances of offering. Chöd uses melodious singing, drums, bells, and horns, and it is generally practiced in locations that incite fear, such as charnel grounds, cemeteries, and remote mountain passes.

dakini (Tib., *mkha'gro ma*). The Tibetan equivalent of dakini is *khadroma*, which literally means "female sky-traveler." "Sky" refers to emptiness, and the dakini travels in that emptiness; that is, she acts in full realization of emptiness, absolute reality. A dakini can be a human woman who has realized her true nature, a nonhuman female or goddess, or a direct manifestation of enlightened mind. Dakini also refers to a class of beings born in the pure realm of the dakinis.

dharma (Tib., *chos*). A very broad term, *dharma* has many meanings. In the context of this book, dharma is both the spiritual teachings that ultimately derive from the buddhas and the spiritual path itself. *Dharma* also means existence.

dharmakaya (Tib., *chos sku*). A buddha is said to possess three bodies (kayas): dharmakaya, sambhogakaya, and nirmanakaya. The dharmakaya, often translated as the "truth body," refers to the absolute nature of the buddha, which all buddhas have in common and which is identical to the absolute nature of all that exists: emptiness. The dharmakaya is nondual, empty of conceptuality, and free of all characteristics. (See also **nirmanakaya** and **sambhogakaya**.)

Dzogchen (Tib., *rdzogs chen*). The "Great Perfection" or "Great Completion," Dzogchen is considered the highest teaching and practice in both Bön and the Nyingma school of Tibetan Buddhism. Its fundamental tenet is that reality, including the individual, is already complete and perfect, that nothing needs to be transformed (as in tantra) or renounced (as in sutra) but only recognized for what it truly is. The essential Dzogchen practice is "self-liberation"—allowing all that arises in experience to exist just as it is, without elaboration by the conceptual mind, without grasping or aversion.

gong-ter (Tib., *gong gter*). In Tibetan culture there is a tradition of *terma*: sacred objects, texts, or teachings hidden by the masters of one age for the benefit of the future age in which the termas are found. The tantric masters who discover terma are known as tertons, or "treasure finders." Terma have been and may be found in physical locations, such as caves or cemeteries; discovered in elements such as water, wood, earth, or space; received in dreams or visionary experiences; and found directly in deep levels of consciousness. The latter case is known as gong-ter, "mind treasure."

guardians (Tib., *srung ma / chos skyong*; Skt., *dharmapāla*). Guardians are male or female beings pledged to protect the dharma (teachings) and the practitioners of the teachings. They may be worldly protectors or wrathful manifestations of enlightened beings. Tantric practitioners generally propitiate and rely on guardians associated with their lineage.

jalus (Tib., *'ja lus*). The "rainbow body." The sign of full realization in Dzogchen is the attainment of the rainbow body. The realized Dzogchen practitioner, no longer deluded by apparent substantiality or dualisms such as mind and matter, releases the energy of the elements that compose the physical body at the time of death. The body itself is dissolved, leaving only hair and nails, and the practitioner consciously enters death.

karma (Tib., *las*). *Karma* literally means "action," but more broadly it refers to the law of cause and effect. Any action taken physically, verbally, or mentally serves as a "seed" that will bear the "fruit" of its consequences in the future, when the conditions are right for its realization. Positive actions have positive effects, such as happiness; negative actions have negative effects, such as unhappiness. Karma does not mean that life is determined but that conditions arise out of past actions.

karmic trace (Tib., *bag chags*). Every action—physical, verbal, or mental—undertaken by an individual, if performed with intention and even the slightest aversion or desire, leaves a trace in the mindstream of that individual. The accumulation of these karmic traces serves to condition every moment of experience of that individual positively and negatively.

kunzhi (Tib., *kun gzhi*). In Bön, the kunzhi is the base of all that exists, including the individual. It is not synonymous with the alayavijnana of Yogacara, which is more akin to the **kunzhi namshe** (see next term). The kunzhi is the unity of emptiness and clarity, of the absolute open indeterminacy of ultimate reality and the unceasing display of appearance and awareness. It is the base or ground of being.

kunzhi namshe (Tib., *kun gzhi rnam shes*; Skt., *ālaya vijñāna*). The kunzhi namshe is the basic consciousness of the individual. It is the "repository" or "storehouse" in which the karmic traces are stored, from which future conditioned experience arises.

lama (Tib., *bla ma*; Skt., *guru*). *Lama* literally means "highest mother." The term refers to a spiritual teacher, who is of unsurpassed importance to the student practitioner. In the Tibetan tradition, the lama is considered more important than even the Buddha, for it is the lama who brings the teachings to life for the student. On an ultimate level, the lama is one's own buddha-nature. On the relative level, the lama is one's personal teacher.

loka (Tib., *'jig rten*). Literally "world" or "world system." Commonly used in English to refer to the six realms of cyclic existence, loka actually refers to the greater world systems, one of which is occupied by the six realms. (See also **six realms of cyclic existence**.)

lung (Tib., *rlung*; Skt., *vāyu*). Lung is the vital wind energy, commonly known in the West by one of its Sanskrit names, *prana*. Lung has a broad range of meanings; in the context of this book, it refers to the vital energy on which both the vitality of the body and consciousness depend.

ma-rigpa (Tib., *ma rig pa*; Skt., *avidyā*). Ignorance. The lack of knowledge of the truth, the base, or the kunzhi. Often two categories of ma-rigpa are described: innate ignorance and cultural ignorance.

nirmanakaya (Tib., *sprul sku*; Skt., *nirmānakāya*). The nirmanakaya is the "emanation body" of the dharmakaya. Usually this refers to the visible, physical manifestation of a buddha. The term is also resonant with the dimension of physicality. (See also **dharmakaya** and **sambhogakaya**.)

prana (See **lung**.)

rigpa (Tib., *rig pa*; Skt., *vidyā*). Literally, "awareness" or "knowing." In the Dzogchen teachings, rigpa means awareness of the truth, innate awareness, the true nature of the individual.

rinpoche (Tib., *rin po che*). Literally, "precious one." An honorific widely used in addressing an incarnate lama.

samaya (Tib., *dam tshig*; Skt., *samaya*). "Commitment" or "vow." Commonly, the commitment the practitioner makes in connection with tantric practice, regarding behaviors and actions. There are general vows and vows specific to particular tantric practices.

sambhogakaya (Tib., *longs sku*; Skt., *sambhogakaya*). The "enjoyment body" of the buddha. The sambhogakaya is a body made entirely of light. This form is often visualized in tantric and sutric practices. In Dzogchen, the image of the dharmakaya is more often visualized. (See also **dharmakaya** and **nirmanakaya**.)

samsara (Tib., *'khor ba*). The realm of suffering that arises from the occluded, dualistic mind, where all entities are impermanent and lack inherent existence, and where all sentient beings are subject to suffering. Samsara includes the six realms of cyclic existence but more broadly refers to the characteristic mode of existence of sentient beings who suffer through being trapped in the delusions of ignorance and duality. Samsara ends when a being attains full liberation from ignorance, or nirvana.

Shenlha Ökar (Tib., gShen lha 'od dkar). Shenlha Ökar is the sambhogakaya form of Shenrab Miwoche, the buddha who founded Bön.

Shenrab Miwoche (Tib., gShen rab mi bo che). Shenrab Miwoche was the nirmanakaya buddha that founded Bön, traditionally believed to have lived seventeen thousand years ago. There are fifteen volumes of biography of Shenrab Miwoche in the Bön literature.

six realms of cyclic existence (Tib., *rigs drug*). Commonly referred to as the "six realms" or "six lokas." The six realms are six classes of beings: gods, demigods, humans, animals, hungry ghosts, and hell beings. Beings in the six realms are subject to suffering. They are literal realms, in which beings take birth, and also broad experiential and affective bands of potential experience that shape and limit experience even in our current lives. (See also **loka**.)

sutra (Tib., *mdo*). The sutras are texts composed of teachings that came directly from the historical Buddha. The sutra teachings are based on the path of renunciation and form the base of monastic life.

tantra (Tib., *rgyud*). Tantras are teachings of the buddhas, as are sutras, but many tantras were rediscovered by yogis of the terma tradition. Tantras are based on the path of transformation and include practices such as working with the energy of the body, the transference of consciousness, dream and sleep yogas, and so on. Certain classes of tantras, of the nongradual transformation path, may also contain teachings on Dzogchen.

Tapihritsa (Tib., Ta pi hri tsa). Although considered a historical person, Tapihritsa is iconographically represented as a dharmakaya buddha, naked and without ornaments, personifying absolute reality. He is one of the two principal masters in the Dzogchen lineage of the Zhang Zhung Nyan Gyud.

three root poisons. These are ignorance, aversion, and desire, the three fundamental afflictions that perpetuate the continuity of life in the realms of suffering.

tiglé (Tib., *thig le*; Skt., *bindu*). Tiglé has multiple meanings depending on context. Although usually translated as "drop" or "seminal point," in the context of dream and sleep yogas, tiglé refers to a luminous sphere of light representing a quality of consciousness and used as a focus in meditation practice.

tsa (See **channel**.)

yidam (Tib., *yid dam*; Skt., *devatā*). The yidam is a tutelary or meditational deity embodying an aspect of enlightened mind. There are four categories of yidams: peaceful, increasing, powerful, and wrathful. Yidams manifest in these different forms to overcome specific negative forces.

yogi (Tib., *rnal 'byor pa*). A male practitioner of meditative yogas, such as the dream and sleep yogas.

yogini (Tib., *rnal 'byor ma*). A female practitioner of meditative yoga.

Zhang Zhung Nyan Gyud (Tib., *Zhang Zhung snyan rgyud*). The Zhang Zhung Nyan Gyud is one of the most important cycles of Dzogchen teachings in Bon. It belongs to the *upadesha* series of teachings.

zhiné (Tib., *zhi gnas*; Skt., *śamatha*). "Calm abiding" or "tranquility." The practice of calm abiding uses focus on an external or internal object to develop concentration and mental stability. Calm abiding is a fundamental practice, the basis for the development of all other higher meditation practices, and it is necessary for both dream and sleep yogas.

Tibetan Works Consulted

Druton Gyalwa Yungdrung (Bru ston rgyal ba g.yung drung), ed. *A khrid thun mtshams bco lnga dang cha lag bcas pa.* Lhasa: Bod ljongs mi dmangs dpe skrun khang, 2009. BDRC W1PD105878.

Lokesh Chandra and Tenzin Namdak, eds. *rDzogs pa chen po zhang zhung snyan rgyud bka' rgyud skor bzhi.* New Delhi: International Academy of Indian Culture, 1968.

Milu Samlek (Mi lus bsam legs). *Ma rgyud thugs rje nyi ma'i gnyid pa lam du khyer ba'i 'grel pa.* In vol. 18 of *Gangs ti se bon gzhung rig mdzod dpe tshogs chen mo*, 381-99. N.p.: 2009. BDRC W1KG14500.

———. *Ma rgyud thugs rje nyi ma'i rmi ba lam du khyer ba'i 'grel ba.* In vol. 18 of *Gangs ti se bon gzhung rig mdzod dpe tshogs chen mo*, 327-45. N.p.: 2009. BDRC W1KG14500.

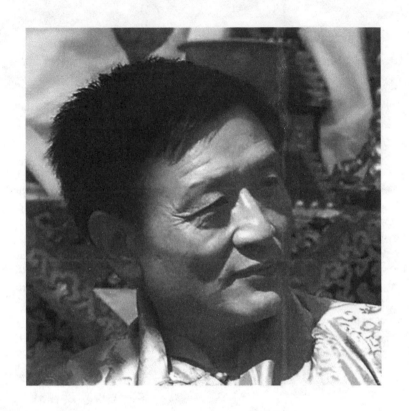

About the Author

Tenzin Wangyal Rinpoche has students in twenty-five countries and teaches in several locations in Europe, the United States, Mexico, Central and South America, and Asia. If you would like information on his and other teachers' schedules, please visit the Ligmincha community website at www.ligmincha.org.